Sharing
Sensory Stories
AND Conversations
with People with
Dementia

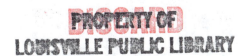

Sharing Sensory Stories
AND Conversations with People with Dementia

A Practical Guide

JOANNA GRACE

Jessica Kingsley *Publishers*
London and Philadelphia

First published in 2018
by Jessica Kingsley Publishers
73 Collier Street
London N1 9BE, UK
and
400 Market Street, Suite 400
Philadelphia, PA 19106, USA

www.jkp.com

Library of Congress Cataloging in Publication Data
A CIP catalog record for this book is available from the Library of Congress

British Library Cataloguing in Publication Data
A CIP catalogue record for this book is available from the British Library

ISBN 978 1 78592 409 5
eISBN 978 1 78450 769 5

Printed and bound in the United States

I see the world more vividly
because I am harvesting the days for you.
Oddities, marvels – something beautiful, something strange.
I collect them for you.
And, sharing them, discover them anew.

Pam Brown, b. 1928

Contents

Introduction

Clinical guidelines from NICE (2006) recommend multisensory stimulation for the management of behavioural and psychological symptoms of dementia. Livingston *et al.* (2014) found sensory interventions significantly improved various forms of agitation. Commentators believe sensory considerations are likely to play a greater role in the care of people with dementia in the future (Behrman *et al.* 2014).

Clearly the sensory world is one to look into when seeking to better support an individual experiencing dementia, but it can be hard for family members, carers and practitioners to know where to start. The whole world is multisensory; what is the difference between the therapeutic use of sensory experience and a person's day-to-day experience of our multisensory world?

This book begins with the fundamentals of sensory engagement work, before going on to explore how sensory experiences can be used in a supportive and enriching way to enhance the lives of people with dementia. It is a practical guide and at every page turn you will find advice and insight to enable you to put what you are reading into practice.

The book is presented in nine sections; each section (excluding the introduction and conclusion) has an orientation and a summary. These introduce the topics covered in the section and summarise them at the end of each section. These orientations and summaries will help you as you dip in and out of the book according to your needs. You may choose to read through the sections in order, and then refer back using their orientations and summaries to pick out relevant information at a later date, or you may choose to jump sections and read those you feel will be particularly pertinent to your current situation. There is no right or wrong way to read this book, do whatever suits you best.

Here is an at-a-glance guide to what you can expect to find in each section of this book:

Section 1 – A note from the author

An invitation from the author to tackle the loss experienced with dementia in a new way.

Section 2 – Sensory engagement and its relevance for people with dementia

Here you will find an introduction to the notion of sensory engagement work, insight into what it looks like in practice and explanation of its particular relevance for people with dementia. This section includes information on how sensory engagement strategies can be used to support someone with dementia to feel safe and secure, to minimise their anxieties and to prevent behaviour problems from arising, these important topics are returned to throughout the book.

Section 3 – The benefits of sensory stimulation

Sensory stimulation holds benefits for everyone, not just those experiencing dementia. In this chapter you will gain insight into how sensory stimulation supports: cognition, concentration, learning, awareness, a person's ability to engage with another person or an activity, mental wellbeing and memory. There are four case studies demonstrating the use of different sensory strategies in the support of individuals with dementia.

Section 4 – Sensory conversations

In order to hold a conversation we need first to be equipped with suitable vocabulary. At the start of this section you will find a guide to seven senses' worth of sensory vocabulary. This information will be a precious resource to you as you move on to constructing some of the simple sensory conversations detailed in the latter half of this section, including sensory exchanges, sensory discoveries and sensory sequences.

Section 5 – Sensory stories

Sensory stories are a wonderful form of sensory conversation, and so versatile in what they can offer to a person with dementia. In this section you will find all the information you need to create and facilitate your own sensory story, as well as a sensory story, 'The Gardener's New Grandchild', for you to try straightaway, together with activity ideas to further engagement with the narrative.

Section 6 – Sensory support

This section looks at:

- how we can use our understanding of sensory vocabulary (Section 4) to enable a person with dementia to retain their independence when carrying out small tasks, and to support them to engage with an activity, either as a part of a group or independently

- how we can use sensory support to set up flight paths to reduce a person's need to express stress through violent means

- how sensory engagement strategies can be used to add satisfaction and enjoyment to a person's life, thus contributing to a reduction of occurrences of distress and violence.

Section 7 – Sensory environments

This section delves into the wonderful possibilities of sensory environments, looking at how we can create our own small (or not so small) sensory spaces for people with dementia. It also looks at how we can assess everyday spaces and make small sensory adjustments to these so that they are more supportive of people with dementia. At the end of this section we look particularly at how carefully thought-out sensory flight paths can be used to avoid outbreaks of violence and how we can create spaces that promote feelings of safety, both for individuals with dementia and for those who care for them.

Section 8 – Sensory support for mental wellbeing

The way we facilitate sensory experiences, especially some of the simplest ones, can have a profound impact on a person's mental wellbeing. Making informed choices between sensory experiences can provide opportunities to support a person's mental wellbeing. Section 7 considers the impact of sensory engagement on mental wellbeing by exploring five concepts that underpin experiences of mental ill health: engagement, time, change, agency and self. We look at how each can be addressed through simple sensory conversations.

Section 9 – Conclusion

We conclude by drawing together all the insights we have shared, and showing how through sensory engagement and conversations, we may continue to maintain a meaningful connection with a loved one throughout their journey with dementia.

Contributors

Coralie Oddy – Reminisense remini-sense.com
Becky Lyddon – Sensory Spectacle www.sensoryspectacle.co.uk
Nina Ockenden-Powell – Wild Happy Well wildhappywell.com
Doug Melia – Safer Handling www.safer-handling.co.uk
Katie Rose White – The Best Medicine thebestmedicine.co.uk

A note from the author

My background as a sensory engagement specialist has primarily been within education and adult care settings. Much of my work has been focused on the life experiences of people with profound disabilities. Often the people I work with have been considered incapable of communicating and learning. My role has been to show how sensory strategies can be used to foster engagement and to facilitate progress which, no matter how small the steps forwards, is always valuable.

Since 2013 my work has also come to encompass the community of people experiencing dementia. As I have carried out this work and (more strikingly, to me) as I have written this book, I have felt the difference between this community and the community of people with profound disabilities. Where I have been used to talking about small steps forwards for people with profound disabilities, with people with dementia we are almost always looking at small steps backwards: skills being lost not gained, and the maintenance of skills, rather than the acquisition of new ones, being the highest aim.

This constant experience of regression is very disheartening. We often speak of it in terms of loss: people lose their abilities and we lose them. Nothing in this book promises otherwise, but I want to encourage readers to approach their thoughts from a different angle.

In times of crisis we learn what matters most. People fleeing war zones don't grab their money or titles as they leave their homes behind, but their loved ones. The nearness of those we love and our feelings of closeness to them are universally more important than any object or any skill we may possess.

My message to people supporting a loved one with dementia is that love and connection need not be lost. Imagine the abilities of the person you are supporting laid out along a line in order of when they were acquired in life. The far end of the line represents that person at the height of their abilities and accomplishments. As we track back along that line we encounter each skill they acquired to get to that point in reverse order of acquisition until at the end of the line, the part of it closest to us, we have only the senses. The person you love is the line. They are there at every stage. You do not lose them as they lose their skills. Your task is to find ways to be with them, to hold them near, to maintain that closeness wherever they are on that line.

The purpose of sensory engagement work for people with dementia is not to recover memories, but to find meaningful ways to be together.

Our struggles come about when we try to connect with a person through skills they no longer possess, for example through the skill of speaking, or through the skill of structuring thought and exchanging memories. Maybe you have opened this book hoping to find ways to help the person you are supporting to keep those skills for a while longer. Sensory engagement can help to maintain skills but that is not the purpose of this book. What I hope you will find in these pages are ways to connect with, understand and support your loved one wherever they currently are on that line, so that, as they travel further into dementia, you can be with them every step of the way. It is not easy and much is lost, but you can still be there with them and that is very precious indeed.

My very best wishes for your journey together.

Joanna

Section 2

Sensory engagement and its relevance for people with dementia

Orientation

In this section you will find an explanation of what is meant by sensory engagement work and insight into its particular potential benefits for people with dementia. We explore how sensory engagement can be used to:

- give someone the opportunity to take part in a conversation that does not rely on words

- combat some of the behavioural challenges that may arise through the experience of dementia

- practically support someone's understanding of a situation or task.

Sensory engagement: a beginners guide

'What is sensory engagement?'

'Isn't everything sensory?'

'Aren't things like this for children?'

I encounter these questions in one form or another frequently as I travel around the country exploring sensory engagement techniques. Often I find that the simplicity of my answers causes confusion, with some people believing complexity is necessary for things to be meaningful or worthwhile.

Sensory engagement is a very literal title; we are looking to engage a person's senses. That is it. I consider an exchange a success if:

- The sense or senses I have aimed the exchange at appear to be stimulated by the stimulus I have offered, and

- The stimulation of a sense or senses leads to an engagement with the person to whom those senses belong.

This act of seeking engagement in a sensory way is something we all do when we interact with one another. You will have encountered the situation of saying something to someone and getting no response, and then raising your voice a little, or calling their name and repeating what you have said, and then getting a response. By thinking of this example in a sensory way, you can appreciate that what you have done is offered auditory stimulation in an attempt to get engagement, and when that did not work you used a form of auditory alert to gain the engagement, and then you offered the stimulation again. On other occasions the person will respond immediately and no alert stimulus is needed.

Of course, talking and exchanging meaning through the use of language is not simply sound, it is also a complex cognitive activity of processing and understanding language – one that is not always accessible to the people we support. Imagine that same communication again, but this time without the language: you offer a sound, but get no engagement, so you offer an alerting noise and then the sound, this time you get engagement. Or perhaps you simply offer a sound and get engagement without the need for an alert stimulus.

What engagement means in the language version of our example is likely to be a reply to a question you asked, or a responsive comment to whatever it was you said. What engagement means in the sensory version of the example comes in many forms. Sensory engagement could be indicated by a person joining in with the experience. So, in our example this would be them making a sound. Sensory engagement can be indicated by body position, facial expression or even a vocal response: someone may turn towards a stimulus, show a response through the emotions portrayed in their face, or even utter a phrase, word or sound in response to the stimulus. Demonstrations of engagement like these are easy to spot. However, in sharing sensory conversations with some people it may be necessary for us to become detectives, spotting their responses from a subtle palette of expressions. It might be that you notice a change in their demeanour that you cannot quite put your finger on. You may notice a relaxing of muscles, a stilling of movement, a certain *something* that lets you know they heard you; they engaged with the sound. When you achieve this, a connection has been made and you have shared in a very simple sensory conversation.

A person's ability to communicate is not dependent on their mastery of certain skills or abilities to utilise traditional forms of communication; it is dependent on our ability to listen fully. We may receive their expression auditorially, but we are just as likely to be listening through other sensory systems as well.

Being attuned to the current way the person you support communicates is critical to their care. We must not rely on or assume that the methods they used to use to communicate are still accessible to them. This sentiment is echoed by researchers in other areas, for example Gerlach and Kales (2017) end their discussion of the importance of identifying pain in people with dementia with the words: 'Simply put, we need to learn the language that our patients with dementia are expressing'. It is our job to learn their language, not their job to retain or re-master lost skills.

Sensory conversations at this fundamental level can sometimes seem so simple as to almost not be there at all, but there is meaning in this passing back and forth of experience. I heard a sound and I shared that sound with you, and you heard it too. That engagement of each of us with the sound is a form of connection. To people unable to access other forms of connection and communication these simple links between one person and another are precious.

There are multiple other benefits to be reaped from sensory stimulation itself which are explored more fully in the next section, but for this introduction what I want to impress upon you is the value of the connection and communication experienced in these incredibly simple sensory moments.

What does sensory engagement look like in practice?

Using sensory engagement techniques could see you offering someone a texture to feel, or holding a light in someone's field of vision. You may find yourself considering the fragrances of bathing products more attentively than before when shopping, or speculating on whether small background noises are confusing a sound exchange you are attempting.

At a more sophisticated level, you may sequence carefully chosen sensory experiences into stories to engage a person in the joys of narrative. You may organise and use a particular set of sensory experiences such that they explain an upcoming event and help a person to cope with it. Or you may arrange an activity, taking account of the sensory presentation of it, such that the sensory experiences that are a part of its presentation support a person in being able to engage with that activity. All of these strategies are explained in more detail in Sections 4 and 7.

When you are taking part in these more elaborate, sophisticated processes, the presence of an 'activity' is easier to identify. You may feel more like you are doing a 'thing'. It will also look more impressive to any onlookers and is more likely to be recognised by observers as an activity, and to be valued. But at the heart of all sensory engagement activities is that fundamental connection through the senses; this is the most important thing and without it an activity (however colourful, smelly, noisy, well-put-together and presented, etc.) is pointless. Sometimes the most powerful forms of connection are the simplest. Although they often seem more impressive, fancier forms of sensory engagement work can risk leaving vulnerable individuals alone in the middle of them if attention is not paid to the underpinning simplicity of the sensory exchanges involved. In Section 4 of this book you will find information to guide you when making choices about stimuli to use for fundamental sensory engagement exchanges.

One of the most wonderful things about sensory engagement work is that its benefits flow both ways within an exchange. Most people undertake sensory engagement work with the hope of offering help and support to someone else, but in the undertaking of it they find that they too benefit from the shared experiences. Someone with later stage dementia may not be able to access typical forms of communication and will need a strategy as pared back as a sensory engagement in order to be able to share a conversation at all. Similarly, someone whose mind has been taken over with worrying about another person, whose day has been full of busyness, can find the simplicity of a sensory engagement exchange invites their mind to slow down for a while, their body to take a pause and to relax. When the facilitator of a sensory exchange also pays attention to simple sensory experiences they are offering, they benefit alongside the person they set out to help. It can be a very equal and rewarding form of experience.[1]

Sensory engagement and dementia

Clearly the opportunity to share conversations in a sensory way is a lovely gift to be able to bring to someone in the later stages of dementia who is no longer able to share in verbal conversations, but actually communicating in a sensory way can hold benefits all the way through a journey into dementia including the early stages. In this chapter we are going to look at some of the primary benefits of a sensory approach for people with dementia.

---

1 Those interested in further exploring the benefits of shared sensory connections may enjoy *Sensory-Being for Sensory Beings* (Grace 2017) which explores how the benefits of mindfulness practice can be facilitated in a sensory way for people of differing abilities.

Communication without the pressure of language

In the early stages of dementia, people are often acutely aware that their faculties are failing them. They make great efforts not to make mistakes and expend a lot of energy masking what can appear to them as their 'failings'. Think of a time yourself when you have been in a situation of stress but were trying to hide your feelings.

Here is an example from a delegate who attended one of my training days. They were tasked with organising a lunch for their boss and some influential figures from other companies. Various things were going wrong with what should have been a simple task: their boss had got stuck in traffic; a dietary requirement had not been met by the catering that had been booked and an alternative needed sourcing to match the food already laid out for the arriving visitors; in the rushing about, coffee had been spilled on their suit and needed sponging off; and so on and so on in an ever escalating succession of small accidents and organisational failures. Whilst trying to fix everything, this person was also expected to engage in small talk with the guests as they arrived. Out of all the tasks loaded on top of them that afternoon, the making of small talk seemed the hardest.

Language places huge processing demands on the brain. To someone already coping with a lot, a conversation can feel like another job on a list that is already getting out of hand. Finding ways to share time and connections that are sensory can be a way to help someone unwind. Partners of people with dementia have reported to me how they find their loved one seems better able to cope, and less troubled by their condition, after an activity that does not require a lot of talking, for example: taking a walk together, getting a beauty treatment together, taking part in a creative hobby, listening to music, or having a massage. Loved ones considering the future of a partner newly diagnosed with dementia may choose to establish a habit of engaging in these sorts of non-verbal activities in readiness for a time when they may be needed.

Choosing a hobby now that can later become a pared-back sensory exchange is a way of creating and maintaining connection through a difficult time. For example, what may now be a weekly walk might in the future become simply sharing together the texture and smells of some plants that grow along the walk you used to take; or the beauty treatment in the spa may become the smell of nail varnish as you paint your nails beside them on a visit to their care home; the craft activity may no longer end in a created product but become simply the touching of clay or the exploring of paint. This sort of progression can be very difficult to think about, and understandably so, but if you do get the chance to consider these topics together ahead of time, that will enable you to make choices about the experiences that heighten the pleasure and enjoyment they offer (e.g. identifying a favourite plant on the walk, or knowing a preferred colour or piece of music). In your discussions, look to identify the sensory elements that you enjoy about the activity as these are the ones that are likely to last the longest for you in your future engagements.

Now, and in the future, being able to be alongside someone without the need for words can be deeply comforting and bonding.

Behaviour and the senses
Oddness

A person with dementia may begin to develop odd habits. For example: staring, getting fixated on a particular item by touching it repeatedly, walking in an idiosyncratic way, and so on. When we try to interpret these actions through our historic understanding of the person, we can quickly become stumped – they just seem odd. But when we understand these actions in a sensory way they can be clues about how their ability to process sensory information is being impacted by dementia. Senses may deteriorate in an idiosyncratic way, or one sense may deteriorate more than another, meaning their ability to work together, which is so critical to our functioning, can be impaired.

As early as 1967, Bower (in Baker *et al.* 2001) described how progressing neuronal losses occurring in people with dementia lead to impaired processing of sensory stimuli, which can in turn make normal stimuli confusing to a person with dementia.

An understanding of sensory engagement work will build your awareness of the sensory world and mean you are more likely to understand behaviours that would otherwise seem odd and be able to sensitively support the person you care for.

Becky Lyddon runs Sensory Spectacle, an organisation dedicated to helping people understand more about sensory processing difficulties. Here she explains how sensory processing difficulties may manifest themselves:

> When someone has a sensory processing disorder their brain finds it difficult to organise and respond to the sensory information it is receiving. The changes dementia causes to the brain can affect how someone processes sensory information.
>
> Someone having difficulties processing sensory information may also struggle with the amount of information they receive. You may see someone overwhelmed by sounds covering their ears, or someone overwhelmed by bright light seeming dazed, or even someone refusing to wear new clothing because to them it is over stimulating. Over stimulation from one or more senses can cause extreme pain, we all respond to pain in differing ways. Gerlach and Kales (2017) remind us that it is important we are aware that a person with dementia may exhibit and respond to pain differently to how we do, and to how they themselves would have done in the past.
>
> Alternatively some people experiencing disordered sensory processing may become really interested in certain sensations and seek out more stimulation. You may notice someone watching how the sun is shining in the room and following how it moves or moving repetitively around whether it is walking or tapping their foot or hand to help reinforce where that part of the body is. These types of behaviours relate to under stimulation from a sense; the person seeks out the stimulation their brain is lacking.
>
> Sensory processing disorder does not mean there is a problem with the sensory organ receiving the information it is the way the brain is organising the sensations.

Distress

At primitive primary level our senses are tools for our own survival. We use our senses to locate food and also to ensure that we do not become food for a predator. In a modern world we also use our senses in many other ways, often in the pursuit of pleasure and entertainment. Sensory signals that would once have meant certain death – for example the visual image of an angry animal running straight for you – may now just mean that we are in the cinema. Yet our senses still retain their primary function: to promote our survival.

Knowledge gained through our senses is prioritised by our brains above all other forms of knowledge. The phrase 'seeing is believing' relates to this, or 'I heard it with my own ears.' Our personal sensory experience is proof of reality and, even when we know we are being tricked, we cannot help but respond. Virtual reality (VR) headsets are a beautiful example of this: a person with a VR headset on knows that what they see is not real, and yet they still duck in response to something swooping towards them, because their senses tell them that it is real. In the battle between the mind and the senses, the senses always win.

The authority of sensory experience is something we all experience. It is not unique to dementia, but for people with dementia it can be more troubling as their sensory systems become unreliable or confused. It is natural for everyone to respond with distress to troubling sensory experiences. If you felt like you were falling, or felt unsteady on your feet you would feel worried, you would grab for things, you would become anxious; it is a natural response to distressing sensory information. For most people, the sensory information they receive about the world matches up to the reality of the world and guides us through it. People with dementia can experience difficulties with their sensory processing, meaning that their senses present them with information that does not reliably portray the world. It is as if dementia is a virtual reality headset that presents a world similar to the one they knew but a fraction more dangerous and distressing.

For someone who feels, essentially, taunted by a confusing sensory world, think how much like a lifeline a clearly-presented, trustworthy sensory experience would be. For people distressed by disordered sensory processing, clearly facilitated sensory experiences can be stabilising and offer reassurance which in turn counters the distress and anxiety they experience in the everyday sensory world. Facilitators sharing sensory stories with individuals with profound disabilities reported a reduction in challenging and harmful behaviour as a result of engaging them in this way (Young and Lambe 2011).

Violence

There is a distinction to be drawn between sensory experiences that disorientate, confuse and undermine confidence and sensory experiences that cause alert or alarm. Whilst the first may lead to a person becoming withdrawn, anxious and frightened, the second can result in violence. This violence is almost always out-of-character with the person as they have been in their life before and is often directed towards people they love and trust. Meaning that, as well as the physical injuries sustained, there are brutal emotional injuries to both parties. Understanding these violent responses in a sensory way can help to avoid situations that trigger them and may also mitigate some of the emotional hurt carers can feel when on the receiving end of an attack.

Before I explain the sensory backdrop that can trigger violence in someone with dementia I want to state a very clear message to those who may be the recipients of that violence.

Whilst what I am about to write may help to take some of the emotional hurt out of the situation for you, I do not want you to feel that you ought not to be offended by being hurt. You are precious. You should not be hurt. To feel okay about being hurt is not right. However much you understand why someone is hurting you, and that it is unintentional or without malice, you must remember your own value. Appreciating your value is a part of being mentally healthy and, ultimately, if you are facing the challenges of caring for someone who may be being violent towards you, it is important not only for yourself but also for them that you stay mentally well. Allow yourself to feel upset by being hurt. Protect yourself. If possible, take time out to restore your balance after you have been hurt.

My father had early onset dementia. On a journey to hospital he tried to get out of the moving car. He required restraining for his own safety. As you care for a person with dementia you may encounter any number of occasions when restraint could keep you both safe.

Often carers are concerned when physical intervention and appropriate levels of force become necessary in the support of their loved one. Even the very word 'restraint' or 'use of force' can strike fear into our hearts. I talk about 'positive handling', 'crisis intervention' or 'safer handling' instead to help people to understand that when we intervene in this way, we do so because we care. Where it has been necessary we should always aim to use the least intrusive and invasive means possible which sometimes can include holding or even just supporting someone and giving them space.

Restraining a person is reasonable when it is both *necessary* and *proportionate* – see Appendix A for an exploration of what these terms mean with regards to physical intervention. Learning effective safer handling techniques can mean that, should you ever need to intervene physically in support of your loved one, you can do so in a way that is effective and safe for everyone involved.

As discussed above, under the heading 'Distress', our senses' primary purpose is the promotion of our own survival. This is, unsurprisingly, something the body prioritises above all else, and this prioritising is evident in the functioning of our brain. You may have heard of 'fight or flight'. This is the brain's response to situations where the senses report danger. In order to promote survival at times of need, the brain focuses its energies on the functioning of the amygdala, the small primitive brain which rests like a walnut at the top of our spinal cord. When triggered, this reflexive part of the brain commands us to fight or to flee. To make sure we stand the best chance of survival, the brain shuts down other processes when fight or flight is triggered; for example it shuts down the ability to process language, to store memories and to retrieve things from memory. More complex thought patterns – like considering the consequences of our actions – become out of reach, as all the energy we have is poured into fight or flight. As with the anxiety responses we discussed above, this is not a response reserved for people with dementia but one common to us all. It is a natural part of being human. It does not represent a failure of character or the revealing of a hidden cruel nature, nor is it born out of previously suppressed resentment or frustration; it is a natural reaction within us all.

What is different for people with dementia is what triggers the response. Whereas a healthy, typically-developed person may have their fight or flight response triggered by sensory information that signals danger, for example if they heard a gunshot sound nearby, a person with dementia may have their fight or flight response triggered by everyday sensory information. This can be exacerbated as sensory abilities deteriorate and become confused by the progression of the condition. Using the information about the senses in Section 4 may enable you to identify and eliminate sensory experiences that trigger violent responses in a person. You can also use an understanding of sensory engagement work to support someone in adjusting their response to what they perceive to be a threatening stimulus.

It is useful to our understanding to recognise that the ordering of the phrase 'fight or flight' is not an accident of language but a reporting of the natural sequence of events. A person whose senses inform them that their life is under threat will respond with violence first; the flight response is second. This makes sense when viewed through the lens of survival. If a predator is threatening me and I am able to employ violent means to kill that predator then I have defeated the threat entirely. If a predator is threatening me and I run away the predator remains a threat to me. Violence is the sensible response of an animal trying to survive – and we are all animals.

Preventing the triggering of the fight or flight response is preferable to developing strategies to cope with the response once triggered. Using the information in Section 4 to identify likely triggers and spending time reflecting on what sensory stimulation the person received prior to becoming violent can help you to identify and eliminate triggers.

It is unlikely that you will be able to prevent all triggers and so you will need strategies to cope with a person's fight or flight response once it has been triggered. These strategies may include the identification of safe spaces for you to retreat to, as well as handling techniques that you can use to keep yourself and the person you are supporting safe, but you may also find sensory engagement techniques can help. In Section 4 you will find information about what sorts of sensory experience are most likely to be calming, and deploying these can help to curtail a violent outburst. In Section 6 you will find guidance about how to support an activity in a sensory way; this same guidance can be used to support and promote flight paths which can then be used to divert a violent fight response into a non-violent flight response.

Consider again that a person in fight or flight mode is thinking with just their primitive brain, their animal brain. Imagine an animal threatened by another animal; for example, a cat meeting an angry dog in an alley:

- The cat senses threat, so its claws come out; ready to fight, its senses do a quick assessment of their situation.

- If the foe cannot be seen, cannot be sensed, then it is likely that the cat will strike out with its claws in self-defence.

- If the foe can be seen, can be sensed, and appears defeatable the cat will attack.

- If the foe can be seen, can be sensed and appears bigger and stronger than the cat, then the cat will turn to flee.

- If there is no flight path then the cat will attack with everything it has, fighting for its life.

- If the foe can be seen, can be sensed and appears equal to the cat, then it could go either way.

- If in that first quick assessment of the situation the cat spotted an escape route then it is possible that it will choose to flee. But if in that first quick assessment of the situation it was clear that there was no escape then it is likely that the cat will attack. Can you see how it is just that tiny window of perceptive opportunity that dictates whether the cat will fight or flee?

For a person it is the same. And often when we try to deal with challenging behaviour we inadvertently do things to exacerbate a situation. For example, we will attempt to move a person's body to turn them away, we will move our bodies to act as a block, we will raise our voices to give instructions. Consider these things through a sensory lens: what signals are sent by touches, obscured vision, raised voices? It is easy to see how, when viewed through the senses alone, these things lose the meaning we intended them to have. The touch becomes the first strike in the attack. The blocked vision means that the person is trapped. The raised voice is akin to the aggressive barking of a dog. They all convey danger – and the response to an increase in levels of perceived danger, is quite sensibly an increase in the levels of violence.

A sensory flight path is a route clearly delineated by the senses that leads to a place of known safety – often this will be a place that offers a low stimulation environment. Again imagine where that desperate cat would run: it would be to a small dark hidey hole – these are the places our senses tell us we are safe. And again it is not just the cat, not just people with dementia, it is all of us. When you are stressed you will naturally retreat to a small space; perhaps you will curl up, wrap yourself up, you will seek out the low level sensory input that you find calming.

Section 6 explains more about creating safe spaces and supporting flight paths.

Sensory support may have a role to play in tackling other areas of difficulty that arise through the experience of dementia. For example, families and care givers have reported inappropriate sexual behaviours as the most stressful and challenging manifestations of the disease with which to cope (Onishi *et al.* 2006). Canevelli *et al.* (2017) observed a strong association between sexual behaviour disturbances and anxiety, leaving open the possibility that actions we could take to reduce anxiety could also reduce this most difficult of challenges thrown at us by the disease dementia. Jakob and Collier (2014) point out that if no suitable activities are provided and people living with dementia have nothing to do, they might become increasingly isolated, frustrated, bored and unhappy. They go on to report the success of simple sensory activities in engaging people with dementia, for example involving people in the sensory aspects of cooking. A finding reinforced by Livingston *et al.* (2014) also found that sensory activities were successful in reducing the agitation of individuals with dementia. More elaborate forms of sensory provision, such as sensory rooms, have been shown to promote positive changes in mood and behaviour in people with dementia (Jakob and Collier 2014; Day *et al.* 2000; Spaull *et al.* 1998; Hope 1998).

Sensory orientation and sensory confusion

Sensory engagement strategies can be used to orientate someone in a setting or with regard to a particular activity – examples of how to do this are to be found in Sections 6 and 7. A person with dementia may find language-based cues for activities or environments confusing and difficult to remember. Being able to utilise a person's senses for orientation gives those who care for individuals with dementia an extra tool in their tool belt of support strategies.

As Becky Lyddon touched upon above under the heading 'Oddness', a person with dementia may experience sensory confusion; it is likely that their sensory perceptions will degrade and that their processing of sensory experience will be altered by the progression of the disease. You will most likely find that the person you care for's sensory perceptions will regress such that they are responsive to sensory stimulation that they would have enjoyed during earlier times in their lives, for example responding to songs from long ago, or reacting to smells from childhood. Their experiences of sensory confusion can become more confusing still if those around them are not aware of what is going on. Section 4 of this book will be particularly useful to you as you try to untangle this confusion.

Grouping sensory orientation with sensory confusion may seem contradictory but actually it is not as ridiculous as it first seems. When we seek to orientate someone through their sensory experiences we are, in essence, giving them lots of opportunities to understand. Instead of just telling them with words we are showing them with images, guiding them with tactile stimuli, supporting them with proprioceptive input and so on. In this book we deal with seven sensory systems; those represent seven different ways to orientate and support a person. Someone who is experiencing sensory confusion in one of their sensory systems will benefit enormously from being orientated through their other systems. And someone who is experiencing confusion through all their sensory systems will benefit from being supported by a carer who knows how to present clear, bold sensory information to maximise their chances of guiding them through that confusion. The information about sensory vocabulary in Section 4 and the advice in Sections 6 and 7 about environments will give you the knowledge you need to be able to offer this guidance.

Summary: sensory engagement and its relevance for people with dementia

Sensory engagement is the practice of engaging one or more of a person's sensory systems with an item of particular sensory interest. Sensory engagement creates a connection between the person offering the stimulus and the individual experiencing it as they both share in a sensory moment.

People with dementia may experience particular challenges to their sensory abilities that mean they are more confused by the world and tasks within it; these challenges can also mean that they perceive danger where there is none. Having an understanding of the sensory nature of these challenges enables us to offer them relevant support, and the later sections of this book look at these support methods in more detail.

Section 3

The benefits of sensory stimulation

Orientation

Sensory stimulation benefits us all, no matter what our age, ability, race, sexuality, gender or any other difference society may choose to bestow upon us. Taking a look at the benefits of sensory stimulation puts us in a better position to understand how providing certain kinds of sensory experiences to an individual with dementia can be supportive.

In this section of the book we will consider how sensory experience benefits:

- the development and preservation of cognition

- concentration and learning

- awareness of a situation or person

- readiness and ability to engage with a situation or a person

- mental wellbeing

- memory.

Sensory experience and the development and preservation of cognition

In our early development our sensory experiences trigger the wiring of our brain. When we receive information through the channels of our senses, this information flies across our brain in little electronic pulses. These pulses leave traces in the brain. If the experiences are not repeated the traces vanish, but if they are repeated then gradually what were mere traces become established neural pathways in the brain, with the synapses connecting to reliably send and receive information.

I have always imagined this as a person walking through a dense forest. The early brain is the densely overgrown forest and a sensory experience is a person walking through that forest. A single experience sends the person treading through the undergrowth once. When we look back at the forest after they have passed the forest is essentially the same, save for a few bent over blades of grass. But if they repeat their journey through the forest many times then gradually their route becomes a muddy track, a footpath, a road, a super highway, an established pathway through the mind.

The more experiences we have, and the more repetition we are exposed to, the more pathways we lay down.

I adore the gorgeous Magic Trees of the Mind images[1] taken from brain scans that show the synaptic connections in the formation of our neural networks at various ages. You can see that in early development the brain's connections are relatively sparse, but as life progresses and more experiences are discovered and re-experienced, more connections are made. In the pictures the pathways are three dimensional; at first there are just a few criss-crossing the brain, but after a while there are more, until we get to two years of age and there are so many paths that the brain is almost completely coloured in.

Think of the forest again: a densely overgrown forest is hard to navigate, how would you know which way to go without a path? But if the whole forest is trodden into muddy paths, then you still

---

1   Diamond, M.C. (2005) *Magic Trees of the Mind.* New York: Plume Books.

do not know which way to go. If everywhere is path, how do you choose which way to walk?

The brain is a clever organ; it knows that having so many channels down which information can flow is not an efficient use of its energies so it begins a pruning process. It cuts the connections which are rarely used or which double up on other pathways. This pruning is conducted against the backdrop of the environment the brain lives in. The messy mud bath of a trampled forest is artfully sculpted into a network of pathways and foliage that perfectly serve the sensing and understanding of the environment it inhabits.

This environmental influence on cognition is the reason why someone who grew up in a busy city may be better able to withstand noise than someone who grew up in the countryside. It is why someone who grew up hearing a language spoken that had no 'r' sound struggles to pronounce the letter 'r' when they encounter it in later life. If you are caring for someone with dementia think about the environment they spent their first few years of life in and use your knowledge of that place to inform the choices of sensory experience you make for them, choosing experiences that are ones they likely encountered during their early years.

What I have described so far is how the brain is wired by sensory experience. If in early life we do not get a rich tapestry of experience we do not create as many pathways through the brain, meaning that when it comes to the pruning stage we have less choice of where we can go; we have to create our bespoke brain based on the routes we have managed to lay down so far.

The opening of the Romanian orphanages in the 1980s gave us a horrible example of what a lack of stimulation in early development can do; we met a generation of children who had grown up without stimulation. The follow-up studies of those children 20 years on show that if stimulation was missed out on after a critical period it could be 'caught up', but if stimulation was missed during that critical period when those initial pathways are laid through that forest then the damage done by that neglect was permanent. Children born with perfectly-functioning minds became permanently profoundly cognitively disabled simply through a lack of sensory experience in early childhood.

Despite the importance of this critical period in the brain's development, the creation of neural pathways is not a once-in-a-lifetime opportunity. The brain is neuroplastic, meaning that it retains its ability to flex and adapt to experience throughout life. Scientists now believe a high degree of neuroplasticity extends until our early twenties and we remain able to lay down new neural pathways throughout life.

It is important that as we grow and develop, we not only lay down new neural pathways relevant to our current experience but also that we allow old ones to grow over. Without the loss of old disused pathways, we would gradually find our neatly networked forest of a brain trampled into an unnavigable muddy field. The process of neurological change throughout life is amazing.

The destruction of neural pathways in the creation of a more efficient mind is to be celebrated, but their degradation and loss through neglect, trauma or disease is very sobering. The creation of those pathways is the creation of our cognition, of our ability to sense the world and make sense of it, to understand, to think, to remember, to communicate. Those pathways, formed in such a simple way – through hearing a sound, seeing a light, or feeling the rain on our skin – *are* our cognition. And those same pathways will grow over and be gone through lack of use and stimulation if we do not continue to walk them. If we find ourselves in environments low in stimulation then our chances of losing our way in that woodland of our mind increases greatly.

As you look to support someone with dementia, you will be looking to give them all the opportunities you can to use the pathways that remain. If they can do a task for themselves, however easy it may be for you to do it for them – and regardless that you might be able to do it quicker or better than them – you will be looking to allow them to do it in order to keep those pathways well-trodden. You will think about the environment they find themselves in: is it one where they feel a range of experiences day-to-day, or one that presents with a dull kind of sensory uniformity? You will find beautiful sensory experiences to bring to them to enable their mind to stay active.

As important as finding beautifully sensory experiences for the person you support to enjoy, is finding ways to enable them to experience sensory feelings of safety.

As you support someone with dementia you will most likely be hyper-aware of some of the pathways through their mind that they are losing. It is easy to focus on this loss, and very understandable. We need also to hunt for the pathways that remain; maybe these paths are not in the state they once were but they still open avenues for exploration and enjoyment to be exploited. Behrman *et al.* (2014) report that for people with dementia, as cognitive function degenerates, the world is experienced at a sensory level, and we can have an influence over the sensations offered.

Trauma and disease are rarely within our power to control, but environment and experience are more readily influenced. Think of the sensory experiences you are encountering right now: what sounds are around you, what colours and shapes, what smells, are you eating anything? Now think of those experiences that you encounter on a daily basis, perhaps the ones you have experienced so far today. They will be countless. Think of the different spaces in which you have encountered these experiences: perhaps inside, outside, in a car, in your own home, in a shop and so on. Count these up over the course of a week and the range is, for most of us, dazzling. Now consider the experiences of someone in a care setting, who may experience the same room, or two rooms, day-in, day-out, for years. Although these rooms may contain different experiences, over time what is encountered is a very limited sensory palette. In such an environment it is very hard for even a healthy brain to retain its capacity, let alone one hampered by a condition such as dementia. In their work about sensory provision for people with dementia Jakob and Collier (2014) report that the deprivation of sensory stimulation and appropriate activity has a devastating impact on wellbeing and health for people with dementia. By finding and sharing even the simplest of sensory experiences with a person with dementia you are helping to counter this deprivation.

As you begin to think about the simple sensory experiences you can use to support a person with dementia, you are thinking about how you are going to support them in their cognitive function. People with dementia experience the world at a sensory level but with reduced ability to integrate and understand these experiences (Behrman *et al.* 2014). How you present experiences is going to affect their ability to process and understand them. Each little experience you find will send a person walking through that metaphorical forest in their brain; the footprints of that person will tread down the undergrowth and help to keep the pathway open. And even if that person encounters a block and cannot get from one end of the path to another, there is still value in them being there. And, who knows? If you send a whole gang of experiences exploring in that confused forest, one or two may just find a way around the blockages that lie in their way. Maybe their footfall will be soft, and the pathways they open up will be temporary, as grass flattened down springs back up masking where they have been, but even still, it is worth it. As you support someone in a sensory way, you may not see a response, but it is still worth it.

We could think of three phases for that forest mind: finding our way, knowing our way and losing our way, and look at what distinguishes these three.

1. Finding our way

At this stage, the forest of our mind was densely overgrown and confusing to the explorer. The first adventurers – those first experiences we had in life – sprang through it full of enthusiasm and relishing their discoveries. The world did not make sense but we embraced experiences and enjoyed walking through the bewildering woodland.

2. Knowing our way

At this stage in our lives, the forest of our mind has been tamed into a neat network of footpaths and foliage. Those who pass through the forest walk with intent: they plan a route from A to B and get there swiftly. In their efficiency, they pay little attention to the wonder of the experience.

3. Losing our way

At this stage in our lives we begin to find pathways we have come to take advantage of blocked or tangled. This is upsetting and frustrating – we feel a loss of power. We know there should be a way through but we cannot find it. We feel distressed. The forest seems scary.

Taking the emotions out of the equation think about how the forest would look during each of these stages. There are a lot of similarities between the first and third stages. The primary difference between these stages is how we feel about our lack of knowing.

In sharing sensory experiences with someone with dementia you are not just seeking to open up routes that were once there, you are seeking to find a way to enjoy the journey through the forest again. You may rediscover memories or find ways around blockages, and those things are very worthy and may be achieved for a short while but in all likelihood attempts to maintain the forest network as it once was are doomed to fail. And if you measure the success of your sensory adventures against such markers you also are doomed to fail. Success is in the journey itself; it is the experience.

In the long term, the more fruitful endeavour is to find a way to enable the person you are supporting to be like those early explorers, delighting in the wonder and the newness. To do this they will need to feel safe. As we progress through this book, as well as exploring how we may find and share wonderful sensory experiences with people with dementia, we will look at how we can use sensory experiences to help them to feel safe on their adventures and enable them to enjoy the landscapes of their minds anew.

Sensory experience for concentration and learning

All of the information we have about the world comes to us through our senses. Our ability to put together information received through different sensory channels is critical to our ability to understand and to learn. In order to learn we need to focus our attention on the information we are receiving; we need to concentrate. At first it might seem simple: the bolder the sensory information, and the more of it we receive, the more likely we are to attend to and concentrate upon it. But it is more nuanced than this. Let us consider a few options; all of the options we will consider have the potential to be right, but some contradict one another:

It will be easier to concentrate on multisensory experience

Imagine the forest of the mind that we have been using as a metaphor. Suppose I am standing on one side of that forest with a message I wish to get to someone on the other side. If I send that message down a single pathway – a single sensory channel – it has one chance of getting through. Suppose that pathway is blocked? My message will not get through. If I can send it through multiple pathways simultaneously then I stand a good chance of the message getting through.

An example from life would be the difference between asking someone to read the message 'stop the horses', compared to asking someone to watch a video of someone saying 'stop the horses' subtitled 'stop the horses', and supported by auditory and visual information coming through on the video showing someone stopping horses.

Clearly a message conveyed through multiple sensory channels is easier to attend to, and therefore concentrate on, and so more likely to lead to learning...or is it?

It will be easier to concentrate on mono sensory experience

Go back to the imagined scenario of me standing on one side of the forest with a message I wish to pass to someone on the other side. This time give more consideration to the person on the other side. If messengers descend on them at once, all urgently trying to get their message across, they may well be overwhelmed and my simple message will be lost in the general babble of all the other messages. Perhaps a message delivered clearly by just one messenger tramping through the forest will be easier to process and receive?

An example from life would be trying to have a conversation with someone in a busy pub: music is blaring, perhaps disco lights are flashing, orders are being shouted to the bar staff, glasses are clinking, the dishwasher is on, the mats are sticky, the beer is sweet, there is the smell of sweat, perfume and food in the air, and your friend is telling you something important. Really important. Are you going to stay put or might you be tempted to suggest you step outside into the cool night air, or retreat to the relative peace of the bathrooms so that you can really pay attention to them? Sometimes less stimulation is a way of getting more information across.

It will be easier to concentrate on sensory experiences presented one at a time

I want you to listen to a note played on the flute. I will play a single note. I want you to listen and tell me whether that note wavers slightly, whether the flute sounds in tune. How would you like me to present this note; how will it be easiest for you to concentrate? Is it in the midst of a song with other instruments playing, whilst we are dancing and drinking, or to truly concentrate would you prefer to sit still with your eyes closed and just focus all your attention on the experience?

All the information we receive comes to us through our senses. How we experience the world is personal to us. For some people a confused background environment would be a busy place full of noise and smells; for other people a confusing background environment can just be their own living room with the sound of the TV in the background. Our experience is always personal to us, and when we are supporting people through providing them with sensory experiences it is important we remember that our experiences are not a guide for their experiences. We have to learn to ignore what our senses tell us is going on and look for clues as to what their senses might be telling them is going on.

Circumstances when it will be easier to concentrate when multiple experiences are experienced at once

I want you to pay attention to me so how do I gain and sustain your attention? If I sit still and offer you just the visual stimulation of my presence, will you notice me? What if I also touch you, so that I am both visual and tactile? Are you more likely to attend to me now? What if I speak as well? And if I am near enough that you can smell me? What if I move so that the visual experience is more exciting?

You are more likely to concentrate on me when I am animated, when I change the pitch and tempo of my voice, when I am bright and cheerful and smell wonderful. Entertainers keep our concentration by constantly changing the sensory experiences they offer us. I will be more entertaining to you when I present myself through multiple sensory channels.

Circumstances when it will be easier to concentrate on a bold/subtle sensory experience.

Think, one more time, of that messenger passing through the brain carrying my message to the person on the other side. If they present that message in a bold way, shouting it loudly and clearly, the person is more likely to take it in.

But think again of who that person is on the other side: suppose they have a terrible migraine. Now if my messenger shouts all that will happen is the sound will amplify their pain and they will cower in agony and not hear a thing. To pass a message to this person I need my messenger to whisper gently.

This translates into how we present sensory experiences in life: are we looking for bright neon colours to engage the sight, or subtle softer shades? Are we going to play the music loud or quiet? Will our touch be a gentle stroke of the hand or a firm grasp of the shoulders?

All of these examples seem plausible in themselves, but they contradict each other. So what is the right thing to do? Are we looking for loud, bright multisensory stimuli that change and entertain, or for single mono sensory experiences that can be softly and subtly presented? There is no one answer to this. We must always to consider the person sharing the experiences with us. Everyone is different and what is right for one person will not necessarily be right for the next. As you expand your sensory practice you will become a sensory detective, working out how to spot the tiny signs in someone's face or body that a sound is pleasing or distressing, or knowing that when a person lashes out seemingly in rage that it might have been triggered by the sound of the car passing outside their room and not by a hidden personal vendetta.

The right sensory experience and the right way to facilitate that experience will always depend on the experiencer themselves.

The diagnosis of dementia gives us a few starting clues for our detective work. We know that people with dementia often struggle to integrate information from their different sensory systems (Behrman *et al.* 2014). In the scenario where I sent the message through the forest with lots of different messengers walking many different paths at once, this message could have been, for example, that I had in my hand a half-eaten pear. The messenger of sight would have said, 'This is green'; the messenger of touch would have reported, 'This is hard, wet and smooth'; the messenger of the somatosensory system would also have reported the firmness of the pear, adding too that 'this is cold'; the messenger of smell would have said, 'this smells sweet' and so on. The person standing on the far side of the forest thinks, 'What is hard and smooth, sweet, wet and fragrant smelling?' and summises that it is an apple. But if they were not able to combine those messages, what they would have received is lots of pieces of seemingly unrelated information. The message of 'I have a pear' would have been lost in a barrage of experience that is likely to frighten and overwhelm.

Being frightened and overwhelmed by confusing sensory experience is not a symptom of dementia, it is a symptom of being human. Imagine being woken in the night to a sound you did not recognise, combined with a weird smell, and a strange sensation on your fingertips – that would be scary. We are all frightened by confusing sensory experiences. Now imagine you live in a flat next door to an experimental jazz musician and above a perfumery: the situation described above would be reduced to simply waking up and wondering why your fingers felt strange. We are all frightened by confusing sensory experiences, but precisely what sensory experiences confuse us is personal to us all.

Present a range of sensory experiences in a targeted mono sensory way covering multiple senses over the course of a communication

For someone overwhelmed by trying to integrate multiple channels of sensory experience you are looking to present experiences in a mono sensory way against a low stimulating background. The experiences you present will target a single sensory system. Of course others may also take in information; for example, someone may see a musical instrument playing a sound, but their seeing it is not critical for their understanding of the experience – the point of the experience is the music. Over the course of a communication you will look to present experiences for different sensory systems so that in an exchange a person has the opportunity to hear, taste, touch, see and so on, but there is never any expectation that they do these things simultaneously in order to be able to access the meaning in your exchange.

Some people will struggle with the multiple sensory experiences in the everyday environment and become distressed by sounds from outside of a room, or people passing through a room. For these people it can be lovely to create a small immersive sensory environment for using reassuring experiences so that they can escape the confusion of their world. Section 7 is about the creation of sensory environments for people with dementia.

Sensory experience and our awareness of a situation or person

In order for us to be aware, we must receive information through our senses. This may seem so staggeringly obvious as to not be worth saying at all. We are so used to our senses working seemingly automatically that it is easy to overlook the process that goes on behind perception. It is also easy to overlook that sensing is not simply a matter of having working sense organs. If we are supporting people with dementia whose sensory perceptions are not working as swiftly as our own it is important that we consider the finer details behind sensing.

For starters, sensation is a two-part process. The first part is the sense organs receiving information about the world and the second part is the brain making sense of that information. We need both parts of that process to work swiftly and smoothly for us to successfully receive information through our senses.

People with dementia may be in later age and be experiencing the deterioration in the sense organs that is common to us all as we age: eyesight is not so sharp, hearing not so keen, taste dulled. This may affect their ability to pick up sensory information from their environment. If someone wears glasses or a hearing aid it is easy for us to remember to make allowances for their perceptual difference, but dementia is based in the brain so there are no outward cues to remind us that perception may be different. Studies have shown that people with dementia may be successfully collecting information with their senses but not be making sense of it with their brains; for example, it was found that people with dementia struggled to recognise and identify odours rather than to detect them (Behrman *et al.* 2014).

Let us think more about this behind the scenes part of sensing, the backstage brain part. Suppose the person you are supporting has perfect vision, perfect hearing, perfect taste, etc. – all their sense receptors are working brilliantly, but they do not seem alert, do not seem to be aware of you or the activity you are offering. What is going on?

All of our senses are active all of the time. Even senses like sight which we think of as being under our control – eyes open, eyes closed – are actually functioning all the time. Close your eyes now, and turn your head to face a light source – you are still receiving visual information. But how the brain attends to and prioritises this information, and which parts of the brain it reaches, change. For example, when we are asleep sensory information is in general monitored by our primitive brain which will alert us to signs of danger but will not take in the detail that higher order parts of the brain used in waking life for perception would register. This waking perception may not happen automatically upon waking for everyone. A person may need to have their senses alerted in order to get them consciously processing information again.

Go back in your mind to those two people on either side of the forest, me on one side sending a message to the person on the other. The person on the far side has fallen asleep, tired from the exertions of the day. I keep sending messages: 'the room is dark', 'there is the sound of rain', but the person on the far side does not wake up. Now suppose that person has fallen asleep not because it is night-time but because they have reached a point of exhaustion. They have received so many messages that they can take no more; they have collapsed at their post. If I want to get a message through now, what I need to do is stop all messages for enough time for them to get some rest and then send a message to inspire them to get up. But what if the person is not asleep, what if they are dazed? All day messages have been coming in, none of them have made any sense and they have fallen into a sort of trance, processing but not attending to the messages. Now what I need to find is a bold 'wake up' message that is easy for them to understand, and hopefully fun, so that when they alert and attend they will be happy to do so.

How does this translate into your practice? Well it may mean that if you are looking to share some precious sensory experiences you will first want to provide some 'wake up' experiences to ready the individual you intend to share these experiences with.

In her book, *The Sensology Workout*, Flo Longhorn (2008) recommends a routine of sensory wake up prior to a sensory engagement session. Having a little routine of seven experiences that address different sensory systems to go through before beginning a sensory conversation is good practice for several reasons:

- The different sensations should serve to alert the different sensory systems of the person receiving them.

- If you go through this sequence of experiences in the same order each time then the routine of the sequence itself, as well as the experiences within it, will come to signal there being something about to happen.

Even if you feel someone's senses are up and running a little wake-up routine like this can help to focus them and create anticipation for the communication to come. A mind prepared to receive a message is likely to take in more information from the message when it arrives than a mind surprised by a message. A sensory wake up routine can be a great way of supporting a person's sensory engagement.

Sensory experience and our readiness and ability to engage with a situation or a person

Our readiness and ability to engage with a situation or a person begins with our sensory wellbeing. Maslow's hierarchy of needs (1943) is a pyramid-shaped representation of our needs; in order to achieve higher level cognitive tasks like concentration we must have our fundamental needs met. Its base level of a safe environment, food and provision for bodily needs applies here too. But we are focusing on the sensory world and so we want to pick apart in more detail what safety means to the senses. Safety is not simply a building that we trust to withstand weather and keep out intruders, feelings of safety run deeper than that.

Promoting feelings of safety at a sensory level requires us to recognise the primacy of sensory experience. A wonderful example of this is our proprioception.

Proprioception is a subconscious sensory system that deals with our awareness of where our body is in space. When your proprioception is functioning beautifully, your awareness of where your body is in space and where your body actually is in space match up. You can test yours now: close your eyes extend your arm to the side of you, point your finger and now bring that finger round in front of your body to the tip of your nose. Did you know where your nose was? And where your finger was? Could you get the two to meet up? Or did your finger land near your nose? Did your fingertip and nosetip align perfectly or were they slightly off? Get a few friends to try – how many of them are successful first time? (Choose these people to be on your team next time you have cause to play pin-the-tail-on-the-donkey.)

You are likely to have had an experience of your proprioception not functioning in accordance to the reality of your life on the boundaries of sleep. Either just as you were waking up, or just as you were drifting off to sleep, you felt like you were falling. That is your proprioception failing to accurately report where your body is in space. You gasp and slap the bed. Not knowing where your body is in space is terrifying.

Pause in your memory in the moment of falling. Your sense of proprioception told you that you were falling. In that moment, in your mind, you *were* falling. Nothing could come between that sensation and you. If I had stood in front of you and told you that you were not falling, it would not have made a difference in that moment because in that moment you *know* you are falling. This is the primacy of sensory experience.

If in that moment I tried to tell you something important, or tried to get you to take part in a fun task, you would not have been able to because that sensation of falling fills your head, heart, mind – your whole being.

What do you do? In response to not knowing where your body is in space you reach, not for verbal reassurance or distraction, you reach for information from another sensory system: you slam your hands to the bed – touch. Your tactile sense reports that you are in fact in bed, and instantly the anxiety of the fall is gone. Now if I stand in front of you and try to say something or offer an activity you are able to engage.

The example above shows clearly how important having a balanced sensory system is for us to be ready and able to receive sensory information. Any one of our many sensory systems can cause us to become unsettled and so less able to connect with and engage with the world around us.

Essentially you will be looking to provide, manage or remove sensory experiences in order to support a person in being ready and able to engage in an activity. It is highly probable that you will need to go through a process of trial and error whilst you work out what sensory modifications best enable the person you are supporting. The four examples below each demonstrate a different sort of provision. These fictional stories are based on facts. Where real people were involved names have been changed.

MAUDE: Offering additional interesting stimulation

Maude was in her early seventies, she had a diagnosis of dementia and lived in a care home. Maude sat in the dayroom of this home every day. Staff reported that she was often agitated, and would vocalise, saying a few words as if about to do something, but nothing that made sense in the context that she was in. Maude would swing her head from side to side as if looking for something or expecting someone to appear. Maude also pinched at her own hands and staff were concerned as occasionally this pinching broke the skin. A conversation with Maude's daughter revealed that when she was younger Maude had been a keen sewer, making her own clothes and fashioning small toys for her granddaughters who were now in their twenties.

Maude was used to being busy, her senses were used to being utilised, yet the home offered a relaxing environment. We all know one of those people who do not find relaxing relaxing! I personally can think of no greater torture than being offered a sun lounger to lie on and do nothing. Maude's agitation at her pleasant environment with its lack of demands of her is not a symptom of her dementia, it is an expression of her self. Where dementia plays its role is in the tasks Maude is now able to do. Where once she would have been able to stitch a zip carefully into a garment, or embroider eyes on a soft toy she is no longer able to do these things.

We created a fiddle blanket for Maude themed around her sewing. It had a zip to do and undo – we stitched a loop of ribbon to this zip so that Maude did not need to pinch her fingers together to operate it but could instead loop a finger through the ribbon. The metal of the zip made a pleasing sound. The zip opened a pocket which we lined with a bright red fabric. Inside the pocket was one of the small toys she had made her grandaughters. The toy was attached by a ribbon to the lining of the pocket so as not to get lost. On another area of the blanket we attached a half-sewn teddy bear head that could be reversed to reveal its furry face. Maude was used to placing fabric right side to right side, stitching and then reversing the stitched item to reveal the fabric facing again. Various other sewing-related items were added to the blanket and it was offered to Maude to have over her knees in the dayroom.

No pressure was placed on Maude to interact with the blanket, but staff and visitors did have a play themselves and show her what to do. We found that for periods of the day Maude's hands would be busy zipping the zip, exploring the toy, fastening and unfastening buckles and buttons. Sometimes she appeared absorbed by the activity and at other times she seemed interested in the room.

Thinking back to that sun lounger – if you give me a book to read I will lie there absorbed in the book; if you give me some crochet to do I will remain there happily and watch the world go by. Maude's fiddle blanket played the same role for her; it enabled her to be at peace within the room and to engage with the room.

For more details about creating fiddle blankets or mitts see Section 6.

GEOFF: Offering stimulation targeted at countering distressing sensations

Geoff was in his fifties, he had a diagnosis of dementia, learning disabilities and autism. He attended a day centre on weekdays where staff found he would often push against other centre users; when taking part in activities he would tip his chair and fidget with his clothing. He did not appear distressed but he did seem unsettled and a member of staff who considered himself to be Geoff's friend said he had always felt Geoff was capable of far more than they were getting out of him.

Difficulties processing proprioceptive information are common in people with a diagnosis of autism so we explored some ways of giving Geoff information about where his body was in space through his other sensory systems. We reasoned that the pushing against other centre users and also the shaking of his body as his tipped chair hit the floor could be providing him with this currently. A weighted backpack seemed to work, but was not useful as it could not be worn for sitting and Geoff regularly lost it after taking it off.

Eventually we found a high-backed chair with firm cushions covered in a plastic fabric. To this we added a wooden beaded car seat cover and also supplied Geoff with an extra cushion which he could use to wedge either between his legs or to the side of them so that the chair pressed against all of his back, buttocks, thighs and hips. We also offered him a beanbag lap tray but found that after using the chair for a little while he did not need this as well.

The chair provided Geoff with a lot of information about where his body was – sat in his chair he no longer needed to seek this information through other more disruptive means.

ROSE: Offering calming stimulation in an attempt to block, blur or mitigate distressing stimuli

Rose was in her late eighties – diagnosed with later stage dementia, she was also receiving treatment for an ulcerated leg which meant that she spent her days in bed. Staff reported that Rose frequently became agitated during the day. At first they had felt this was in response to pain from her leg but an increase in pain medication had not had any effect. Descriptions of Rose's agitation fitted with both pain and fear.

Rose was not able to tell us what was distressing her, and the pattern of her distress did not give us any useful clues. We speculated that something in the environment might be alarming her – perhaps a noise, a smell, the pattern of light, we did not know. If we had been able to work it out, perhaps we could have changed it. But as we could not work it out we instead sought to create a personalised sensory environment around her bed that would be calming for her. We hoped that if she were calm she might be better able to cope with one of the experiences that worried her if she did encounter it. We also hoped that by creating the environment we might block out the negative experiences, whatever they may be, and that if they were pain related then the stimulation offered by the environment might distract from any physical suffering.

With help from Rose's nephew, a large shelf bracket was fixed to the wall above her bed; from this we were able to drape two plain white shower curtains, creating a canopy effect. Matched sensory experiences are more reassuring than mismatched ones so we found a simple sound responsive colour changing light that would enable us to match the visual stimulation we were offering Rose with the auditory stimulation of her favourite music. The colour changing light was placed on her bedside table together with a speaker and a lavender scent diffuser. The home were happy for us to erect our improvised tent during the day when Rose was frequently viewed by staff who passed by her open bedroom door regularly, but asked that it be taken down at night for reasons of safety.

We showed staff how to pull the curtains forward and tie them with bits of ribbon stitched to the corners, to Rose's bed so that Rose's view became almost completely curtain with just a triangle of the real world at the foot of her bed. Rose's nephew downloaded some of Rose's favourite music onto a mobile phone that could be connected to the speaker. He chose tracks he felt would be calming. The music could then be played and the sound responsive light switched on, meaning that from within her bed tent Rose heard her favourite soothing melodies, smelt lavender and was treated to a gentle display of colour changing lights on the sheet canopy.

We did not want Rose to miss out on the life of the home around her so we agreed with staff that she would spend time in her makeshift tent for an hour in the morning and another in the late afternoon – these times were chosen as they were when staff felt that Rose was most likely to be agitated.

Staff were asked to record when Rose was agitated before the curtains were erected and after, however high staff turnover and shift working meant that very few staff actually noted down incidents of agitation so our assessment of whether this little improvised sensory environment had been successful was largely based on word of mouth. Several months after we had created the tent Rose's nephew reported that she had become agitated during a visit and had seemed to grab at the curtains. He had taken this as a request and pulled them around her bed and Rose had calmed. We believe that we created a safe place for Rose to retreat to when she needed it and to spend time in regularly to top up her reserves of coping for the rest of her day.

For more details about creating improvised immersive sensory environments see Section 7.

DAVIDE: IDENTIFYING AND REMOVING DISTRESSING STIMULI

Davide was in his mid seventies and had recently moved in with his son and daughter-in-law after having several accidents at home requiring treatment in hospital. The family suspected that Davide might have dementia, reporting that some of his behaviour seemed out of character and erratic.

After sharing afternoon tea with the family a video camera was set up to record Davide as he prepared his evening meal. The family were keen that Davide maintain his independence despite living with them and so had organised that he would prepare his own meal early in the day at a time when he was used to eating and then sit with them and have a hot drink whilst they ate their evening meal later.

Davide appeared to flinch from time to time whilst making his dinner, and as the task continued and small mistakes in the preparation were made he became more frustrated and more hurried in his actions. It was clear to see how this combination of rushing whilst frustrated could lead to accidents.

After repeat watchings of the recording we speculated that Davide was flinching at sounds in the environment around him. Certainly he flinched at the doorbell and at a phone notification from a phone left in the kitchen. Smaller sounds like a cupboard slamming and the sounds of the children playing in the room upstairs also appeared to bother him.

Davide had moved from a home where he lived on his own to a busy family home – anyone doing this would find the transition difficult, but where someone functioning on all cognitive cylinders might be able to identify the cause of their frustration and challenge it by asking for some peace and quiet Davide seemed to not quite understand it and so was buffeted by it in a way he clearly found upsetting. His frustration was not directed towards the cause of his agitation but towards himself for not being able to sort it out.

Simple adjustments were made to the home and to the habits of the people within it. A shoe rack by the front door prompted the children to swap shoes for slippers or bare feet, making their footfall on the floor above the kitchen softer; the doorbell had options for different tones and a softer tone was selected; the loud cupboard had small rubber dots stuck inside the door, and everyone tried to remember to either turn their phones to silent or vibrate or to choose softer notification sounds.

On a second visit the family were delighted with the adjustments. Davide still seemed on edge but it is always difficult to tell from the outside how a person truly is. The instincts of loved ones are to be trusted. It may well be that although we had eased Davide's transition from quiet home to noisy home a little he was still experiencing low levels of distress and confusion caused by his dementia.

Sensory experience and our mental wellbeing

When we are mentally well we think outwardly: we notice the world around us, pay attention to the people in it, make plans for a future and look forward to what life may bring.

When our mental wellbeing dips (the mental health equivalent of having a cold) we think inwardly: the world around us passes us by; the people in it are a blur and the future is to be feared.

Perhaps when feeling down you have heard one of these two very irritating phrases 'Smile! It could be worse' or 'Wake up and smell the roses.' Unfortunately what makes these phrases all the more annoying, and their smug pronouncers all the more justified in their smugness, is that they are both in fact good advice: when we smile the physical act of smiling releases hormones in our brain that make us feel happy.

Similarly when we engage with our sensory experiences it takes us out of ourselves and brings us into the present. Mindfulness is the practice of paying non-judgemental attention to the present. Mindfulness has been shown to be preventative of stress anxiety and depression and to slow down telomere decay and, in so doing, slow biological ageing (Epel *et al.* 2009). Fostering connection with the sensory world around you is a good way to add a little dose of mindfulness to your day.

Of course we also get pleasure through our senses and attending to pleasurable sensory experiences is a way of boosting our mental wellbeing. But the experiences need not be especially pleasurable to be mindfully explored. Simply notice the texture of the seat on which you are seated, feel the weight of this book in your hands, and notice the sensations your body is receiving.

Think of your memories of sensory experiences. Do you remember handling warm pebbles, or laying your palms flat against hot tarmac in the sun, or the feel mud between your fingers, sand between your toes, fists of torn grass, the feel of cold water as you swam? What age are you in these memories? If it is more than five years younger than you are now, put this book down immediately and go out and update that age. Stop and smell the flowers – actually do it – update your memory banks – yes you know what those things feel like but make time to feel them anyway. Live richly through your senses. Indulge them every chance you get. Joy and calm will follow.

Scent is an important form of stimulation to provide when looking to support mental wellbeing in a sensory way. Our ability to smell and our mental health work closely together, such that an engagement with scent can have a positive impact on our mental health and mental ill health can affect our ability to smell. This is because our sense of smell is processed by the limbic brain, the part of our brain that deals with emotion and memory, whereas our other senses get processed by the thalamus. Later on in this book we will talk about the importance of not overwhelming people with aromas and how to go about choosing smells for people who may be suffering from mental ill health.

Mental ill health can affect our ability to use our senses to receive sensory information from the world. By providing someone with simple sensory experiences we are inviting them out of themselves, away from their worries, their anxieties and fears, and into the present to the experience we offer. And in finding these experiences, in harvesting the sensory world for the person in our care, we support our own mental wellbeing as well. Beyond the simple provision of these experiences, how we allow them to unfold and to be interacted with can further support a person's mental wellbeing. For example, in the story above Maude felt a loss of her sense of self in an environment where she was expected to relax. Maude's self-esteem through life was founded in her usefulness to others, her busyness was her identity, and the opportunity to be busy once more was to reconnect with her sense of self and her self-esteem. As we explore examples for sensory activities you will be able to link them all back to mental wellbeing.

At the end of this book, in Section 8, you can find insight into how to facilitate simple (or more elaborate) sensory experiences to be supportive of mental wellbeing.

Sensory experiences and our memory

At the start of this section I took the metaphor of a forest to represent the brain. Some of the pathways through that forest are our memories, and some of them are how we get to our memories. As the forest changes so our ability to remember changes and our memories may vanish or become cut off from us; the information about what happened to us is still in our minds but out of reach. Keeping the pathways of the mind well-trodden can help us to maintain our memories and our access to them.

In a book about dementia memory is always going to be a big topic, but this book is not about memory. A person is in part their memories, but only in part – when memories are lost the person shaped by those experiences and their continuing experience remains. This book is about the person as they are today, so in this section I will focus on two things that relate to sensory experience and memory: how sensory experience can be used to support our memory and how memories can be shared through sensory experience.

First, let us look at two types of forgetting: state dependent forgetting and context dependent forgetting, and the role of sensory experience in these.

Context dependent forgetting is when you walk out of a room, forget why you walked out and only on returning to the room do you remember. We have all done it. What prompts your memory are the sensory experiences within the room. You are reminded by the sounds, sights, smells, etc. of that room. In studies researchers found people better able to remember information in the context in which they had learned it.

In terms of the person you are caring for this may well mean that they are able to perform certain skills, access certain memories, know certain things, in the context in which they learned those things. The memories we laid down during the time when our mind was most neuroplastic, those from early childhood to our early twenties, are often the most durable. Revisiting places where these memories were created can be a way of uncovering knowledge.

Often times people with dementia will need to move home. This move, from a place where they knew what to do to a place that is new to them can be very disabling in terms of their skills and abilities. There are ways to mitigate for this: having care at home, or moving into a care setting as early as possible would help but they are hard to achieve. The second best option is to try and create a sensory continuity between the home the person is familiar with and the new home. Can you use the same wallpaper? The same colour of paint? The same laundry detergent? Can their kitchen utensils move with them? And so on. Think of all of these things on a purely sensory level – think in terms of sights, smells, sounds, the tactile experiences on offer. Even a few familiar items can help a person to feel secure and in feeling secure and safe they will be better able to engage with their new setting.

State dependent forgetting is like context dependent forgetting but instead of the physical context you are in, what is changing is the chemical state of your body. The chemical state of your body is effected by all sorts of things, many of them sensory; for example, the light levels in the room, how much sleep you have had, what you have eaten or drunk, medications you have taken, how stressed or calm you feel and so on. As with context dependent forgetting a person is better able to remember when they are in a similar chemical state to when they took in the information.

In terms of the support you are offering a person this may mean that you look to share a particular activity always at the same time of day to enable them to get as much out of the activity as possible.

The most important thing to recognise with memory and learning is that when the brain is stressed memory and learning cannot take place. If a person is being stressed by their sensory environment this will prevent them from accessing their memory banks and could lead to them seeming more disabled than they are. A stressed brain shuts down the centres that process emotion, learning, memory in order to focus all of its energies on survival. When a brain does this the person that brain belongs to enters fight or flight mode. The person may become very violent or run away, and it is important that as the person caring for this individual you do not take this extreme behaviour to heart. Remember their emotional centres are shut down; in that moment they cannot feel. It is likely that they love and respect you a great deal, but they have been separated from their ability to access these emotions and knowledge by the stress of the situation.

Summary: the benefits of sensory stimulation

Sensory stimulation is critical to the development and preservation of our cognition. Understanding how sensory experiences can be confused by the deterioration of neural pathways in the mind can give us insight into how we can adjust how we present experiences so that they are easier for a person with dementia to process and understand.

Sensory stimulation affects awareness, engagement, concentration and learning; being aware of how different sensory influences can affect a person's ability to do these things can help us to put in place supportive stimuli or withdraw disruptive stimuli.

Sensory stimulation plays an important role in mental wellbeing with an engagement with the sensory world being good for our mental health. This effect goes both ways with poor mental health impairing our ability to engage with the sensory world. How we can support mental wellbeing through sensory engagement work is further explored in Section 8 of this book.

Finally, sensory stimulation has clear links with memory, and well chosen sensory stimuli may connect a person with their memories.

Section 4

Sensory conversations

Orientation

If we are to have a conversation we first need vocabulary to populate that conversation with, so this section starts with insight into what constitutes sensory vocabulary for seven sensory systems. For each system we consider the sensory experiences that are most likely to gain a response from a person with dementia.. We consider how you can judge what might be most appropriate for the particular person that you support and also how to ascertain what sorts of reactions you are likely to get to a stimulus (e.g. will it be calming or exciting). Once we have our vocabulary in place we move on to some simple sensory conversations. Sensory conversations do not need words, they can be the simple sharing of an object or the more elaborate revealing of an object or set of objects. In latter half of this section we look at some different ways of structuring sensory conversations.

Communicating through sensory experience

What we think of conversation is hugely bias by our use of language. When we acquire language it changes the way information is stored in the brain and alters how we view the world. People who use language often experience the world second hand through their linguistic understanding. This was beautifully articulated to me by a delegate on one of my training days: Andy Edmeads, a hospice worker who shared a poem he had written about his own sensory reflections with me (an excerpt is below). I love his phrase, 'I am a citizen of the secondhand' – I think this is how many of us lead our lives and the invitation to engage with the sensory world that comes to us through a desire to support someone in a sensory way is an invitation to live first hand once more.

Immediate or second hand?

I don't know why I bother to watch
Match of the Day
Commentators tell me how my team have done
Analyze every mistake, every move
Tell me why my team hasn't won
I did love that Argentinean Tango
But the judges show me where the hold
was wrong, the steps out of time
And the film critic explains the deeper meaning
I have missed
Even the bird watchers guide book
Tells me where and what to look for
Habitat, markings, flight
And I am no longer surprised
by colour and movement
Instead I look for distinguishing marks
And give it a name
I am a citizen of the second hand
Receiving life through the screen
Of other peoples' perceptions
The experts tell me who to vote for and why
I cannot make up my own mind
I gave it away some time ago
But those darling little boys
Citizens of the immediate
Show me another world
Of wonder
first hand, wide eyed

they drink it all in
They open my eyes once again
To the immediate, to real presence
Restore to me, my lost infancy
Performing life, first hand...

A conversation is fundamentally the exchange of meaning between two parties. We can elaborate on this and say that the exchange of meaning happens in a turn taking way and that the meaning is sequenced and structured. But essentially we are looking at the transference of meaning from one party to another. Words are little parcels of meaning, but they are not the only way it can be expressed. Our bodies express meaning as they move. As children we all knew what it meant when an adult stood over us, their hands on their hips, a frown on their forehead. No words were necessary, we understood! Similarly, when you smell the warm rubber of a hot water bottle, or the scent of a particular meal baking, it means something to you. Sensory experiences carry meaning and when we share these with each other we have sensory conversations.

If we are to have sensory conversations we need first to equip ourselves with some vocabulary. Having an understanding of what sorts of sensory experiences will best suit the person you are supporting is akin to choosing the right language for a conversation. In the following section you will find an insight into sensory vocabulary for seven sensory systems.

Sensory vocabulary: great sensory experiences

We are looking for sensory experiences for our sensory stories and conversations that are attention grabbing, sense filling and relevant to the experience of the person we are going to be offering them to. Below you will find a consideration of what these might be for each of seven of our sensory systems: visual, auditory, olfactory, gustatory, tactile, proprioceptive and vestibular.

Visual experience

Our society is hugely sight dominated and the ability to take in information visually is assumed in nearly all contexts. Because we are used to using our vision to access the information around us it is easy for us to think that an interesting visual experience is an informative one; for example, a picture with a lot of detail. However when we are looking for sensory experiences we must focus on the sensory aspect and not associated meaning which may require certain cognitive skills to access.

A picture is only an interesting visual experience if you understand that pictures hold meaning, and also understand what meaning you are looking to get from that particular image, and even then it is only interesting if your eyes work well enough to pick out the small details. If you do not understand these things or if your eyes are not as good as they used to be then it is likely that a picture held out as a visual experience will be a splodge or two of colour of little interest at all.

When we consider what makes for a good visual experience we want to think of things that really grab the eye. A funny but rather effective little test you can do to locate things of visual interest in a room is simply to shake your head and try to allow your vision to blur as you do this; as you confuse your visual field a few things will stand out – most likely the bold block of light coming from the window and any particularly bright object in the room. These were the things that still ignited the interest of your vision when your understanding of what you were seeing was confused.

Attention grabbing visual experiences are likely to be bold bright blocks of colour presented against contrasting backgrounds. Consider using neon colours which give off more light than typical colours. The contrasting background is important, when you shook your head to pick out the points of visual interest in the room those that contrasted with the background were the ones you spotted. Because vision is the processing of light by the retina the more light someone is asked to process, the bigger demand is placed on their brain and the more easily they can be overwhelmed. For this reason if you are hoping to get someone to look at a particular object, presenting the object well lit against a dark background is your best chance of gaining their interest. If you hold an object up for inspection in a brightly lit room it is likely that there are any number of other visually interesting things around that their attention may be drawn to. It is also possible that all the light will tire out their willingness to attend to visual information and they may become unresponsive to your attempts to engage them in sensory conversation.

Super simple supportive resources

- A lovely simple resource to have to support visual engagement is a piece of **black cloth** with a matt finish (shiny surfaces present a confusing visual experience because of their reflective nature). This cloth can be placed over a table or on someone's lap and be used as a background to the visual experiences you are offering.

- **Small pen torches** enable you to add more light to an object, the brighter an object is the more information is received by the eye about it and so the more visually interesting it becomes. Pen torches enable you to pick out an object from its background and illuminate it. It is also possible to buy UV pen torches. UV light turns non-visible light into light the eye can process; things that fluoresce under UV light give off nearly 20 times as much light as ordinary objects so a UV pen torch can be a terrific tool for boosting visual attention.

- **Coloured cellophane** provides a different sort of interesting visual experience. So far in the examples described above we have been looking to locate a single item in the visual field and have that be one of significant visual interest. With coloured cellophane you can facilitate a big visual experience for someone but one that does not require them to look in a particular direction. When we look through coloured cellophane everything we see changes in its appearance so it is a big visual experience. Sunglasses and magnifying sheets (sold to help people read small print) do the same thing – sunglasses would be a great visual experience to accompany a story about a holiday in hot climes.

All of our senses follow a line of development. For most of us we progress a long this line so quickly that we barely notice it happening. But as we lose our sensory abilities we tend to lose them in the order in which we gained them, with those skills we learned first remaining with us for the longest, and those we learned more recently fading first from our repertoire. If you are supporting someone whose sensory skills are leaving them, as is the case for many people with dementia, having an understanding of what these early developmental experiences are can cue you in to experiences that may still be accessible for them. If you are curious to know more about these early developmental sensory experiences my book *Sensory-being for Sensory Beings* has chapters detailing the development of each sense and options for interesting experiences to stimulate each of seven sensory systems.

Early developmental sensory experiences are often the ones that remain accessible to people with dementia when other experiences from the same sense have faded. I call these beacon experiences.

Visual beacon experiences

- **The colour red.** You may find that an individual with dementia is better able to identify objects that are red in colour; consider using bold blocks of red to gain or focus people's attention. A Dementia Cafe local to me has found that food served from red plates got more attention than food served on white plates. Presenting red against a natural green background is a lovely way to make it accessible.

- **Black and white images.** Sight is a two-part process: the first part is the receiving of information by the eyes and the second part is the making sense of that information by the brain. The clear contrasting messages of black and white are much easier for the brain to decipher than subtler messages like peach and lemon yellow.

- **Faces.** Our eyes are hardwired to look at faces: we do so reflexively. The face reflex in our eye is triggered by the slightest representation of a face; it is why we see faces in clouds and in abstract patterns or ink blots. Just a line drawing of two eyes and a smiling mouth will trigger the face reflex and gain our visual attention.

If you are planning on using your own face to gain visual attention, or indeed if you are planning to hold out an object to gain visual attention, it is worth considering where best to position yourself or the object. Most people's vision naturally settles at a distance that is about elbow length from their own face (their own elbow) so you are most likely to gain the visual attention of someone not currently attending by holding an object up to them at this distance directly in front of their face.

Having an understanding of where best to position your face to get attention can be useful when greeting people. For example, if you are visiting someone in a residential setting it is likely that you walk in to find them seated. Your head is high up; theirs is low down. What we typically do is begin our greeting once in earshot. So the seated person hears a voice, but does not necessarily see a face. To present a clearer greeting we can wait until we have either sat down or bent down so that our face is clearly visible and then say hello and who we are.

Auditory experience

Sound surrounds us all the time; in order to listen we have to pick out one sound from other. Our ears get pretty good at doing this over a lifetime but this skill of discriminating between sounds can be lost. It is also often disrupted by the introduction of hearing aids which amplify *all* sounds, not just the ones we want to hear. Someone getting hearing aids for the first time must re-learn how to discriminate between sounds. If their brain is struggling with other things this re-learning may be hard to do. And if their brain is already struggling with confusion and hearing aids are introduced the sensation of being swamped by sound can be very distressing.

When offering auditory experience to be attended to we are looking for a sound that will be easy to spot amongst all the others, for a clear presentation of that sound at a loud, but not too loud, volume. Part of your consideration of what sounds might be interesting is a consideration of the pre-existing background noise. Where will you be sharing this sound experience, is it somewhere with lots of traffic noise? Or a crowded environment with lots of language around? Hearing words around other words will be harder to do (for anyone) than hearing words against a sound back-drop of rustling leaves or quiet music.

Different types of sound are processed in different locations in the brain, so you may find someone responds more to one type of sound over another. It is worth exploring what sorts of sounds a person responds to positively as you look to select sounds for your sensory conversation. As you will know already music and singing are wonderful ways of eliciting response to sound.

Beacon auditory experiences

- **White noise sounds.** Ssshhing noises are likely to be soothing to people: the noise of a hair dryer or a vacuum cleaner, the whir of an engine, the buzz of a refrigerator – these are all white noise sounds which we find easy to process and comforting. White noise will also mask other small sounds like clicks and pings that might otherwise alert and alarm us.

- **A person's name.** Our name is one of the sounds we have heard most frequently through life; it was one of the first words we understood, and our brain finds it very easy to handle it. When I am meeting a friend for a chat I might not say their name at all, I will greet them with a hello and we will chat away together and say goodbye having not spoken our names at all. But if I am meeting a friend with dementia I will try to say their name as often as possible. In doing this I am offering them a friendly sound experience that connects us together; the sound of their name is pleasant to them, it connects them to impressions of memories of people who knew them and cared about them, and that I am a person who knows their name means I am a person who knows them. That word alone conveys our friendship and our connection. If my friend is in a care setting where they maybe encountering staff who do not know their name I will want to see if I can find a way of letting people know their name so that they are able to use it too and my friend feels connected to the people caring for them. I will look to share their name in the form in which they prefer to be addressed (e.g. whether they prefer to be addressed by their first name alone, a nickname, or more formally). There are lots of ways of doing this, jewellery or clothing can be worn that is personalised with a person's name. Perhaps my friend could have a personalised mug, or their room will display cards that have their name on the front of them. It does not need to be much, just having their name written somewhere near to where they are will enable people meeting them to use it to connect with them.

Laughter

Laughter is a wonderful sensory experience and holds a lot of other benefits, as Katie Rose White from *The Best Medicine* explains:

> Laughter is universal, we learn how to laugh before we learn how to talk, it is integral to the bonds we make in infancy and continues to help us relate to each other as we get older. As well as these social properties, laughter has an array of amazing health benefits. It is a natural stress reliever reducing levels of cortisol in the blood; it improves physical and mental wellbeing and has been scientifically proven to increase our tolerance to pain.

> 'The health sustaining factor may not be laughter itself but how laughter and humour are used to confront life's challenges' (Provine 2000, p.199).

> Learning how to laugh even when you do not feel like it can be an incredible coping strategy, like Provine suggests it is our willingness to laugh when faced with challenges that is the real power. When we laugh (whether real or fake) the physical act releases feel good endorphins around the body transforming our mood and allowing the weight of the day to be alleviated.

If we choose to respond positively to life's little blips then we can be mentally more prepared and resilient when bigger challenges head our way.

Katie Rose White is a laughter facilitator who runs workshops across the UK helping participants to manage stress, panic and anxiety through the use of simple but very effective laughter techniques. Experiencing dementia is often stressful and worrying for all involved, and seizing any opportunity to laugh together and to include everyone in that laughter can only be a good thing.

Tactile experience

We are continuously receiving tactile experience, therefore to be noticeable a touch experience must stand out against the experiences already being processed. Think about what you are touching now (until you read those words you were not attending to these sensations) perhaps you can feel the fabric of your socks, your clothes, the pressure of a chair against your legs, the feel of the paper at your fingertips. None of these tactile experiences were holding your interest until your attention was directed to them by my words.

We attend to the tactile experiences that stand out from the ones we are currently in receipt of, so in a world of fabric we notice the piece of grit in our shoe. If you are looking to interest someone in touching an item consider how similar it is to the things they are already touching and hunt for an experience that will offer a contrasting sensation.

Because so many tactile sensations are being received by the touch organ (our skin), if we are looking to engage someone in a tactile experience we are looking for one that will be noticed. Presenting a bold experience is one way to get attention. Touch experiences that are hard, sharp, rough, cold, etc. all present bold messages to our tactile receptors. Clearly some of these can also be dangerous but you can find ways of facilitating experiences like this safely (e.g. a nail brush is both hard and spikey whilst also being safe to explore).

One of the fundamental purposes of touch is to keep us safe – our skin is constantly on alert ready to sense when something that might harm us touches us. This is why we tune out the pre-existing touch experiences; it is important that we learn to ignore the sensation of our legs against the chair so that we are better able to respond to that small tickle of a spider beginning to climb our leg. When you offer someone a touch experience it is likely that their attention will be drawn to it in the first instance but will then fade as that experience becomes a part of their background tactile experience. To maintain attention we need to find ways of facilitating touch experience such that it keeps happening (e.g. instead of placing the nail brush against someone's hand, move it around a little in a continuing fashion).

We can take advantage of how big the touch organ (skin) is; other senses rely on much small sensors (e.g. sight and the eyes). Often touch experiences are offered to the hands, which is a shame as there are so many other places touch can be explored. Think about where on the body has a lot of nerve endings, these places are places where more touch information will be processed and the reverse of this is places on the body with relatively few nerve endings where touch information will be muted.

If you are supporting someone who seems particularly sensitive to touch then offering experiences to less sensitive areas (e.g the skin of the upper arm) can help them to be willing to engage with them. Likewise if you are supporting someone who is finding it difficult to attend to a touch sensation then offering them the experience to a sensitive area of the body (e.g the soles of the feet or the mouth) can help them to register and engage with the experience.

Using the mouth to explore tactile experience is a very sensible thing to do – we have a lot of nerve endings on our lips and because they are soft and squishy it is easy for us to shape them around objects and explore them in detail. As we learn to use our touch we find out tactile information about objects with our mouths and use this information to inform our understanding of what we feel with our hands. If our hands become less sensitive or information comes through to our brains in a muddled way, a very sensible strategy for us to use to stay informed about the tactile world is to put things in our mouths. This can be dangerous and it can be frowned upon. Those supporting individuals with dementia need to ensure that the objects available to them are safe to be explored with their mouth if they are likely to do so. A person employing their mouth to back up their information about touch is a person actively addressing difficulties presented to them by their dementia, a person still engaged in exploring and understanding the world, a resourceful individual doing a very sensible and pragmatic thing in response to a challenge they face – this is a person to be respected not frowned at.

Beacon tactile experiences

- **Deep pressure touch experiences.** Light touch experiences are processed by the skin alone, but when pressure is added to touch the deeper tissues of our body also respond. Deep pressure touches are things like hugs and handshakes, shoulder squeezes – these touches are innately reassuring and comforting. It can be easy to approach people with dementia with gentle touch – often people in later age appear fragile and to give them a bear hug can feel a bit much. Light touch is one of the hardest touch experiences for us to process and if our sensory abilities are disrupted for any reason, light touch can even be painful; it can feel sharp, a little bit like being electrocuted.

- If the person in your care is indeed too fragile to be the recipient of a firm hug then finding alternative ways to offer touch experiences that stimulate deeper tissues will be useful. **Massage** is an obvious answer – simple hand, foot or shoulder massage sequences are easy to learn and can be wonderfully connective and calming. For a more unusual solution try using a large inflated ball (physio balls are great for this) or balloon to roll over the person's body, applying pressure as you go (e.g. a beach ball could be rolled up someone's legs and over their lap with pressure applied as a part of a sensory conversation about going to the beach).

- **Nurturing caring touch** has physical and mental health benefits. Many individuals with dementia are the recipients of a lot of functional touch, as people help them with daily tasks and attend to their personal care needs, but very little nurturing caring touch. Nurturing caring touch is any touch that is intended to show affection or care but that has no functional purpose (e.g. a goodbye embrace, a hug, a handshake, a reassuring hand on the shoulder). These sorts of touches are part of our bonding with one another and sustain relationships and feelings of connection. This much we know intuitively already, but what is perhaps more interesting is that research shows that nurturing touch can have physical health benefits (Kulkarni *et al.* 2010).

- Studies done on neonates demonstrated that **containment holds** had particular health benefits. Clearly this is research done on tiny babies so it may not generalise to the rest of the population but it seems reasonable to presume that if something is beneficial to the health of ones so medically fragile that it might also hold benefit to others as well. Containment holds are things like hugs that contain a person. Some people can find hugs overwhelming and medically fragile individuals may not be able to safely receive hugs or may be positioned such that hugging them is tricky. What the scientists found with the neonate research is that it is possible to facilitate the health benefits of touch with other less intrusive containment holds (e.g. one hold involved placing one hand on top of the recipient's head and then using the other hand to cover both of the recipient's hands – these would be placed one on top of each other on their tummy or lap so that they could both be covered by the hand of the person delivering the hold). Using this type of hold with an individual with dementia could be a lovely way of telling them that they are cared for whilst also providing the physical health benefits of nurturing touch.

Touch and emotions

Our emotions are conveyed through our touch. Touch is an essential part of bonding and communication for everyone, not just for those individuals who are sensory communicators. For this reason it is very important that we are mindful of our own emotions when facilitating a touch experience for someone who cannot access all the forms of communication we access.

If I am stressed and I touch you I will convey that stress to you through my touch. If you are also able to understand my words and I tell you that I have just had a particularly difficult time in traffic coming to see you, you will understand that the stress you felt in my touch was to do with the traffic and not with you. Someone not able to access the extra information through other channels will just feel the stress and will not understand why.

If you are a member of staff working in a dementia care setting it is important you reflect on your own emotional state as you touch your clients. It may be that there are days when because of difficult circumstances in your own life you are not best placed to offer touch to the people you are supporting and you may need to ask a colleague to step in instead of you.

If you are caring for a loved one with dementia and feeling stressed you are much less likely to have someone you can hand over to in times of need. What it is important for you to remember is that caring for yourself is not something that should come second to caring for your loved one. In fact caring for yourself is a fundamental part of caring for your loved one and should come first. If you do not care for yourself you will not be able to care fully for them. You are not being selfish by attending to your own needs, you are being responsible. You are not letting them down by taking time out to wind down, relax or have fun, you are putting the resources in place that are needed for their care. Without doing these things you will not be able to care in a meaningful way regardless of how much you care emotionally.

Touch policies

All settings that support individuals with dementia should have a touch policy that details what touch is for and how it is used and who should be delivering it within that setting. If you work in such a setting you should have been asked to read this policy when your job began and you should be familiar with it and use it to inform your day-to-day practices. If you support a loved one with dementia who accesses care in a setting you should ask to see their touch policy and be ready to offer your feedback on its appropriateness for your loved one.

Sadly there is a history of these policies being written in the negative, detailing touch that is not allowed and discouraging people from touching one another. Often such policies are based on the entirely false notion that preventing touch prevents abuse. Let us be clear: preventing touch does not prevent abuse. Preventing touch makes abuse more likely. Preventing touch dehumanises people, making it easier for people to treat others as if they are objects.

Of course inappropriate touch should not be used and a touch policy will want to mention this, although to be frank if a person is willing to touch someone in an abusive way it is very unlikely that the wording of a policy is going to have any affect on them and the idea that someone could accidentally touch someone in an abusive way is pretty absurd. We all know instinctually what touch is appropriate and what is not, it should not need to be said, but of course a policy can state it. But this is not what a touch policy should be used for. A document that just states the obvious is not a helpful document.

Touch policies should give the message that touch is acceptable and should detail the different forms of touch, how they are used and why they are used, including a wide range of nurturing touch. Staff should feel empowered by a touch policy to offer nurturing caring touch to those in their care. When staff feel confident offering caring touch and work in a setting where that is encouraged they feel a greater job satisfaction as well as providing a better standard of care.

An individual with dementia may be facing a lot of personal distress and fear, they can be confused, frightened, anxious. For any of us if someone near to us was feeling in that way our natural response would be to offer comforting touch. Language is difficult for the brain to process; it is difficult to follow and be reassured by language when we are stressed, but touch is wonderful. People reflecting on difficult times in their life will talk about the person who was just with them, who didn't say anything, who just sat beside them, put an arm around them, held their hand and got them through it. To not offer this sort of touch to someone in your care who is in need of it is abusive, it is neglect.

Gustatory experiences

Taste experiences can be fun to offer as a part of a sensory conversation. You are not looking to provide someone with a whole meal, just a little nibble to accompany your conversation. For those who cannot nibble, taste can come through fluids or even through things such as flavoured lip balms.

You may be thinking that the gustatory world offers a wonderful range of experiences to choose from but actually, if you are accessing taste experience alone, it is very limited. We taste just five flavours: sweet, sour, salty, bitter and umani (a savoury flavour). We only access all the other flavours when we use our sense of taste in conjunction with our sense of smell. As our sense of smell tends to degenerate through life many people with dementia who are in later age will have significant impairment to their sense of smell which will in turn mean that eating is really rather boring. How excited would you be by your food if there were only ever five flavours available to you?

If you think that the person you support may be finding eating dull, you can look to invest it with sensory interest that they can access through their tactile and somatosensory sensory systems (e.g. by providing food that is: hard, crunchy, chewy, hot, cold, runny, thick, food that melts or even food that explodes or bursts, as is the case with things like popping candy or simple rice crispies or cherry tomatoes).

Beacon gustatory experiences

- **Sweet experiences.** Nearly all of us has a sweet tooth and sweet flavours are likely to be enjoyed by all. Finding sweets that people enjoyed in early childhood is a great way of garnering a positive response.

- **All the rage experiences.** Find out what foods were 'all the rage' when the person you are supporting was in their late teens and early twenties. It could be that these were food products that were new on the market at this time or were considered the luxury treat of the day.

- **Novel experiences.** As well as finding taste experiences likely to connect people with positive memories it is also good to choose experiences that have no expectation of memory tied to them so that you offer the person you are supporting the chance to express their opinion as who they are today and to be valued in the current moment. Brand new novel taste experiences are a great way to do that and are a good equaliser; you can all try something new together.

- **Hot and spicy experiences.** Because people with dementia often experience impairments to their olfactory sense it is likely that the person you support will be accessing a reduced palette of taste experiences. Taste experiences of heat, that is not temperature but rather the hotness of spicy foods or pepper, are actually processed by the somatosensory receptors that enter our face along our trigeminal nerve. These sensors are responsible for sensing temperature and also pain. The sensation that we associate as the taste of spicy food is actually processed by our somatosensory sense and not our gustatory sense. This means that although not strictly a taste experience we can offer someone a different taste when we offer them this type of sensation.

Olfactory experiences

Our sense of smell is unique among the senses, being the only one processed by our limbic brain, our emotional brain. All of our other senses get processed by our thalamus, our thinking brain. Because of this smell packs a big emotional punch and smell experiences that connect to memories are likely to transport people in time back to moments of heightened emotion (fortunately these are often positive memories).

Because of the different way olfactory experiences are processed it is very difficult for us to conjure up smells in our thoughts, therefore if you are looking for smell experiences to share with an individual with dementia it is important that you get out there and sniff things. You will not find smell experiences by thinking about them, you have to go hunting for them. We tend to think of food and drinks as giving off smells, which of course they do, but they are not especially smelly things, they are just the things we hold close to our nose on a day-to-day basis. Hold other things there and you will discover they smell too.

Thinking a little bit about how smell works can help us to facilitate more powerful smell experiences and indeed to support those individuals mentioned above when we were discussing gustatory experiences who may find their olfactory experience diminishing.

The process of smelling takes place inside the nose where scent molecules in the air get dissolved against the mucus lining. Because the molecules need to be dissolved it is important that anyone seeking to access olfactory experience is well hydrated. Having a blocked nose due to a cold or needing a nasal oxygen supply will also affect a person's ability to smell.

Assuming we are well hydrated in order to smell we need scent molecules to be present in our nasal cavity. Holding things close to the nose means the molecules they are releasing are more likely to enter our nose. Sniffing briskly is not helpful to accessing olfactory experience as this draws those scent molecules past our smell receptors super fast, giving us very little time to process them. A better approach is a slow steady inward breath through the nose. If sharing a smell experience with someone this slow steady breath is something you can model; most people will naturally copy what you do.

Increasing the number of molecules available to the nose is a good way of boosting olfactory experience. Two simple ways of doing this are:

Keep smells sealed inside plastic tubs; the scent molecules released will all be caught inside the tub meaning that when you open the lid there will be more molecules in the air to be accessed. So, for example, if you are using essential oils as a smell resource (these are super as there are a huge variety of scents available and they're very cheap) you will get a bigger experience from a few drops of oil left on a cloth or cotton pad stored inside a plastic pot than you will from simply opening the bottle and sniffing the neck.

Heat is a form of energy; when energy is added to a substance it excites the atoms making them move about faster and the faster they go the more likely they are to break free from the object and become scent molecules in the air. If you think about smell memories you have they will often relate to hot places or times (e.g. summer heat waves, hot holidays, fires, baking). Warming anything up will make it smellier.

Types of smells

We actually have two types of smell receptors in our nose: ones that register the volatile scents – these are the things we typically think of as being smells (e.g. the scent of flowers, of hot tarmac, of soup being cooked, of perfume) – and ones that register pheromone scents. Pheromones do not smell in the way we typically use the word smell. They are not smelly! But we do pick them up through our smell receptors and respond strongly to them. We might not notice ourselves doing this but the pheromone markers of the people nearest to us are extremely important to us. The pheromone smells of our nearest and dearest are deeply comforting to us and the pheromone scent of our partners is hugely significant in our choice of mate; we are very unlikely to mate with someone whose pheromones do not complement our own. These people will be the ones we see as attractive but just do not fancy.

Beacon pheromone olfactory experiences

- **Baby's head.** Babies between the ages of 0 and 12 weeks give off a very strong pheromone smell from the top of their heads to encourage us to bond with them. Clearly this is a very tricky experience to facilitate without the aid of a newborn baby but it is one worth noting just in case someone you know should happen to have a baby and to visit.

- **Primary carers pheromones.** The pheromone scents of those closest to us are very comforting to us. If you are supporting someone with dementia it is very likely that you are supporting someone who is in need of a great deal of comfort. If you are their nearest and dearest your pheromones will be comforting to them, and doing simple things like sleeping on a newly washed pillow case a few nights yourself before moving it onto their bed, or letting them hold a T-shirt you have recently worn, are all ways of giving them access to your pheromone scents without you being with them. Of course they will also be able to access these comforting scents when you hug them or are nearby.

- These comforting scent experiences can, with a little bit of planning, also be facilitated for people in care settings. The 'smell noodle' detailed in this Facebook photo album http://ow.ly/uMds30c5Jq0 is one option. Another option that would be relatively simple in practice but would take an open and understanding conversation to set up would be to speak with the person who is closest to the individual with dementia, this could be their partner or their children or whoever is their closest loved one, and see if you can set up a pillow case exchange. If that person was willing to sleep on a pillow case for a few nights and then seal it inside a ziplock bag to preserve the scent they could bring it to you and you could use it on the bed of the person in your care, or they could even hold and hug the pillow at times of need. You are not asking someone to bring in a dirty smelly – as we understand the word – pillow case; it should not pong but just from having had them sleep on it, it will have acquired those precious pheromone scents and so offer a comforting olfactory environment to their loved one. Of course the scents will not last very long so you would need to have a few pillow cases so that they could be rotated.

Beacon pheromone olfactory experiences

- **The laundry powder from home.** Find out what laundry powder the person you are supporting was used to using at home; this smell will be associated with their own clothes, their freshly washed bed linen, their towels all those home comfort things. Laundry detergents often have quite strong smells so suddenly being surrounded by a different one can be quite alienating and disorientating.

- **Perfume of the era.** Work out what the favourite perfume or cologne was when the person you support was courting. Typically this will be the fragrance that was all the rage when they were in their late teens. Even if it was not a scent they wore themselves they will have smelt it when out and about looking for love. Of course if you know what scent they themselves wore that will be brilliant.

- **Parents toiletries.** What soap was used at home when they were a child? What was their mother's hand cream? What was their father's shaving foam? Asking these questions of a person with dementia whilst they can still answer you is a great way to store up sensory conversations to have in the future when words may not be such effective tools for communications.

- **Baby care.** If you are supporting someone who had their own children then the odours associated with early childcare (yes, all of them!) can be positive olfactory conversations to have. These can be especially meaningful conversations for children to have with parents with dementia. If the child rubs a little of the baby lotion their mother used to use on them as a child into their mother's hand and their mother responds to that smell. Perhaps she pauses and stills as she smells. In that response is a message for that child that says, 'I am your mother, I remember caring for you'; it is not as articulate as the verbal message but the meaning is there in the recognition of that smell.

- **Smells associated with good times.** What was baked to celebrate festivals significant to the person you are supporting? Were candles lit? Was incense burned? Did they go to a place that has particular smells associated with it?

Go on some smell adventures together; see what you can find. Be careful though, because as smell is processed by the emotional brain it is very easy to overwhelm people with odours. Stick to just a couple per sensory conversation and save others for chats another day.

As well as providing an interesting source of sensory conversation smell activities have added mental health benefits. Actively engaging in smelling is good for your own mental wellbeing, as well as the mental wellbeing of the person you are caring for. Having someone to look for smells for can be a good motivator to get out there and smell things yourself. We are funny, in that when our cognitive capacities are fully functional we tend to miss out on activities through our presumed knowledge. We look at the flowers in our garden and know they smell nice, but we do not actually go out there and smell them. If you actually go and smell them, if you pause in the supermarket to sniff the different brands of shower gel – if you lift things up to your nose and smell them – this has a positive impact on your mental health. What a wonderful side effect of hunting for sensory resources.

The flip of this is that if you are experiencing poor mental health, that will have an impact on your ability to access stimulation through your sense of smell. People with depression are less able to receive scent information than people who are mentally healthy. If you are supporting someone who may be feeling this way, or indeed if you yourself are feeling this way, then what you are hunting for is a smell to break through the malaise. Something bold and bright and zingy that you will be able to register and maybe take interest in. Try a scent like peppermint or lemongrass.

Proprioceptive and vestibular experiences

Your proprioceptive sense tells you where your body is in space. Close your eyes, extend your arm out to one side and point your finger. Now bring your fingertip perfectly to the tip of your nose. Perhaps you miss; perhaps you are able to get it right first time. The sense you use to perform this task is your proprioceptive sense, you use your awareness of where your nose is combined with your awareness of where your fingertip is to unite the two.

Your vestibular sense tells you whether your body is in motion or at rest and whether it is balanced or not. It is the one that tells you when the aeroplane you are in takes off – even if you have your eyes closed, you feel yourself tip backwards.

Both of these senses can be impaired. They are subconscious senses so sometimes they are not viewed as being as important as our famous conscious senses but they have just as big a role to play in our understanding of experience and engagement with the world. To have these senses impaired or confused is debilitating and confusing. To not know where your body is in space is to feel as though you are falling and to not be able to understand motion and balance is to feel seasick and fall over.

The information we get from these senses is only meaningful to us if it is partnered with information from another source; for example, we may know where our hands are in space but this is of little use unless we also combine it with the visual information of where the glass that we want to pick up is located. Movement partnered with a strong source of information from another sense is a great way to stimulate these senses, and a great example of partnered proprioceptive and vestibular stimulation would be to dance in a room where there was a strong light source (e.g. a window) or a strong sound source (e.g. speakers in one corner).

Beacon proprioceptive and vestibular experiences

- **Rocking** is a very soothing proprioceptive and vestibular experience – very stressed individuals will often rock themselves. There is a school of thought which suggests we ought to stop them from doing this for fear they will appear weird to outside observers, but the logic of this is somewhat puzzling. A person rocking in response to stress is taking responsibility for calming themselves down; to block them from doing this is likely only to make them more stressed and the next step in this sort of self-soothing behaviour is likely to be some form of self-harm. If we are worried about a person rocking we should seek not to stop the rocking but to sort out whatever is the source of their stress. It maybe that the source of their stress is not something we can solve, in which case we might turn our attention to looking at how we can help them to cope with it, they have already made a start with their rocking and it is time for us to join in. Can we work out ways to help them be rocked, maybe ways in which we can be there with them? We cannot rescue them from their stressful situation but we can be with them through it. What about a swing bench where we can sit side by side and rock gently? Or a hammock? Or what about taking time out at intervals through the day to dance a little, to rock side by side gently together? If you are able to offer a person with dementia the experience of rocking at regular intervals throughout the day you are offering them little moments of calming. Presenting rocking in this way: little and often can help them to maintain a calm state, rather than waiting until pressure has built up to such an extent that they feel the need to shut down and just rock on their own.

- **Spinning** is a big source of stimulation to the vestibular sense and can be a lot of fun. Often we do not like to be spun too much, but the odd spin here and there is joyful and exciting. Dancing is again a wonderful way to do this. If you are supporting someone who is a wheelchair user consider whether spinning their chair might be something they would enjoy. Of course if you spin around too much you can knock yourself out; there are very few sensory experiences where this is the case so we need to be careful. Spinning one way and then the other to counteract the rising of the fluid in our inner ears is a good precaution to take.

- **Wrapping, brushing and massage.** People who are struggling with their proprioceptive input experience a very unnerving sensation of not quite knowing where their bodies are in space. One you have probably experienced on the boundaries of sleep is where you momentarily felt like you were falling. Feeling like this creates a lot of anxiety and fear so experiences that counter it are very reassuring. Any experience that gives you big pieces of information about where your body is in space will counter unnerving gaps in your proprioception. Some examples of things you might do for people in your care are:

  - Offer them massage; the tactile experience of massage gives information about where our bodies are.

  - Stroking someone's skin with a brush with relatively rough bristles. As you stroke along the skin you map out where that body part is, larger brushes can be used to give bigger pieces of information.

  - Being wrapped safely but securely gives tactile information about where our bodies are in space. This could be a shawl around the shoulders or a stretchy piece of fabric that it is possible to fit one's arms inside. You may find the person you care for is comforted by sleeping in a sleeping bag or even sitting in one so that their legs are enclosed.

A note about balance and vestibular input

It is common for people in later age to experience little falls. It can mean that they are processing the information from their vestibular sense less well and so they are overbalancing more frequently. It is important that we go about supporting them in a way that will make them less likely to fall, not more likely to fall, and how we do this is slightly counterintuitive so it is easy to get wrong.

The intuitive response to falling over is to be more careful not to fall in the future. But because our vestibular sense is a subconscious sense our subconscious mind is the one skilled at interpreting its messages. If we concentrate on balancing we ask our conscious mind to take over a process it is not skilled at administering and consequently we are more likely to fall again. In order to support someone who is struggling with their balance we need to encourage them, not to focus on their balance but to focus on the partnered experience that goes with their balancing. Think about people who are experts in balance, like high wire walkers, these people do not focus on balancing, they focus on looking. Their concentration is on the visual experience that informs their vestibular experience not visa versa. Providing bold sensory cues as to where a person is in space can help them manage their subconscious senses (e.g. outlining door frames in a bright colour) or ensuring there are bold visual messages about orientation in a room (e.g. a bold dado rail).

Simple sensory conversations

Now you have your sensory vocabulary you can begin to engage in some simple sensory conversations.

Sensory exchange

The most basic conversation you can have is simply sharing a single sensory item. Perhaps as you were reading through the sensory vocabulary section above a particular item stuck out to you and you wondered how the person you support would respond to such an item. That is a great place to start: find the item and share it with the person you are supporting. People can worry about how to introduce smelling something, or touching something. 'What do I say?' You do not have to say anything, remember words are something you find comforting, they may not be comforting to the person you are supporting. At other times a very short verbal intro can be all that is needed, 'Look what I found', and then let words fade and explorations take over.

You do not need to push someone to take part in a sensory activity. You can explore the item yourself and then offer it to them to copy your explorations. We naturally follow another person's lead in this way, and you can follow their lead back. For example, you might be sharing the smell of some soap rubbed into a facecloth.

You pick up the cloth and hold it to your nose and take in the scent, then offer it to them for them to do the same. Naturally they copy your movements and smell the soap; you leave the cloth with them and they begin to toy with it with their fingers; you can reach out to it and do the same, perhaps your joining in with the movement will make them pause; you take the cloth back with a smile and pull it over the back of your hand feeling its texture with your skin, then hold it out to drag across the back of their hand. You can see how an exchange like this has the natural to and fro of conversation and if done with a glint in the eye contains a lot of playfulness, and friendly connection.

The description above is of a pure exchange, an object chosen only for its sensory properties and explored jointly as a conversation that is purely sensory. You can of course have a conversation like this around an object that refers to another place, event or time (e.g. the soap smell in the example above could be the smell of a particular soap from a particular place in that person's life.) When sharing a referenced sensory exchange many facilitators hope that it will bring memories to the surface, and indeed it might. But remember that these can be there whether words are there or not. So in the playful sharing of the smell of soap from a time long ago you may be joining that person as they play in their memories, dancing in and out of a flickering recollection of another place. You may choose to refrain from putting language into this situation, knowing that if you do you place a processing demand on their brain that may cloud out the joy of the moment you are sharing and bring them back to a present where they are aware that their capabilities are fading. This can be more about your own abilities to manage yourself than to manage them. We badly want to know what another person thinks and feels, especially if that is a person close to us. When we see a glimmer of a memory in their eyes we want to reach for it and share it too, to say 'What is it? Do you remember?' to offer prompts. Try and just enjoy the glimmer – maybe it is real, maybe it is not. But if it is, then you can be in that moment with them, like sitting in a patch of sunlight as clouds momentarily clear. Do not worry about understanding precisely what the light means. Just enjoy the feeling of it and the togetherness in it.

Sensory discovery

Another very simple sensory conversation to have with a person is a discovery conversation. This sees you discovering a sensory object that is concealed in someway beforehand, or revealing an aspect of a sensory object that was at first not apparent.

Think of how we normally go about sharing a story with a friend. We rarely reveal its content straight away, and if we want to play with them or increase interest in our story we may begin it with phrases such as 'You'll never guess what happened…' or 'Did you hear about…?' These are our little verbal ways of adding tension and suspense, they increase the pleasure we experience in sharing stories. We are also liable to add twists to our stories as they go along, again to make them more entertaining and enjoyable – and to show off a little to the people around us! A sensory discovery conversation is the sensory equivalent to the above and a great way to add a dimension to a sensory conversation to make it that bit more interesting, mischievous and fun, it is almost like the sensory equivalent to gossiping!

For all of these you will begin with your choice of vocabulary, choosing a sensory item to hide or reveal that you believe will be of interest to the person you are sharing the conversation with.

- **Handbags.** Have an item hidden inside a handbag and open the bag to reveal it. Other sorts of bags would, of course, also work.

- **Boxes.** People naturally associate a box with wondering what is inside of it; finding boxes that have particular sensory appeal will add to this effect (e.g. boxes that are an unusual shape or boxes that are brightly decorated). In the case study in Section 5, Coralie Oddy from Reminiscene describes how she used a parcel to ignite interest in an activity.

- **Cloth coverings.** A tea towel laid over an item on a tray, a lightweight piece of fabric draped over items on a table, all provide for that dramatic magician whipping a table cloth away sort of reveal.

- **Two-sided items.** Pictures with a mirror on the back, reversible fabric, fabric with reversible sequins, etc.

- **Cards.** Like boxes, people are attuned to open a card, or an envelope, and small flat sensory items can be hidden inside.

- **Peg bags.** These are cheap to make or buy, easy to store as you can hook them onto a rail or string, and fabulously versatile as you can keep all manner of things hidden inside them.

If you work in a care setting what about preparing a range of sensory conversations to offer to people who visit, a bit like a good dinner host preparing some conversation starters for a formal party?

A sensory sequence

A sensory sequence is another layer of complexity in our sensory conversations. Here, as we sequence sensory experiences, we are mirroring the ordering of our words in a typical conversation. The sequencing itself holds meaning on top of the vocabulary within it. In a verbal conversation this sequencing is necessary for the conversation to work at all. As I can demonstrate by repeating this sentence without its useful sequencing: Can I repeating by this without its as demonstrate useful sequencing sentence!

With a sensory sequence the sequencing itself is not fundamental to the success of the communication but it still adds a layer of meaning to the exchange creating a more sophisticated conversation.

Sensory sequences can also be thought of as the sensory equivalent to a sentence written down that can be read back independently when a communication partner is not present. Think of how you might leave a note at someone's house if you visited when they were out, or how you might write a note on a postcard to share a moment from your holiday with a loved one far away. In creating sensory sequences we can pass sensory notes to our loved ones for them to enjoy in their own time.

To create a sensory sequence you need a length of string or a washing line. Many shops sell travel washing lines for as little as a pound and these can be ideal as they are sold complete with pegs. If you are using a piece of string I recommend buying some small bulldog clips or small carabiners to use with the string. Hang the string along a wall or length of fence. Make sure the space around the string is clear from trip hazards. You can use a washing line strung across a garden but this can make it difficult for people to balance whilst accessing the resources. Ordinarily in an environment we use our awareness of things like doorways and steps and walls to navigate and maintain our balance. Because we hope to focus the attention of our explorer on the resources we will attach to the line it is likely that we are also going to distract their attention away from these naturally orientating cues in the environment, therefore it will be very helpful if there is a wall or sturdy surface nearby for them to steady themselves against.

Once you have your line fixed in place you will be looking to clip along it various items that each have different sensory properties. Often taste experiences are missed from such an experience but there are plenty of ways of hanging up a little snack for someone to taste. I have seen people use miniature gumball dispensing machines to add sweets to a sensory sequence, but things like lollipops or candy canes are easy to hang and by using a hook for a hanging basket you can suspend a plate with anything on it that you wish. You might choose to theme the experiences on your line so that they all relate to a particular topic. Cultural or religious festivals work well as a source of inspiration as often they incorporate a wide variety of sensory experiences. Aim to cover as many senses as possible with the items that you suspend from the line.

Another set of experiences that can be tricky to include are sounds – of course there are various things you can hang from a line that will jangle and rattle and these will be super if they fit the theme of your line, but for more specific sounds we need an alternative. One option is to use talking tin lids – these are sold to support people with visual impairments in understanding the contents of the tins in their kitchen cupboards but can be put to much broader use than that. They are about the size of a tin lid, and often they are magnetic or sold with a strap which means they are easy to attach to stuff. You can record samples of sound onto them very simply and the sounds you record will be played back at the touch of a button. If you use them regularly the people exploring your sensory resources will get used to pressing the buttons to discover the sounds.

You can explore the line with someone or leave them to explore it at their own pace, as if it was a note that you had written to them.

Some people will struggle to walk along a line hung against a wall or along a fence; for these people you might look to create a line you can move to them. You can buy metal clothes rails relatively cheaply; these are super for turning into a sensory sequence as items can be hung from them tied to coat hangers. They have small wheels on the bottom to allow them to be easily moved around so one could be wheeled up to a person's chair or bed for them to explore. A smaller and even simpler alternative is to create a mini sensory sequence on a coat hanger, this can then be hooked onto something in front of the explorer (e.g. onto the back of another chair). A regular coat hanger will fit three or four sensory items hung from its long edge.

Here are some example resource lists for sensory sequences about different topics.

A train ride

- A whistle to blow that sounds like the train whistle.

- Travel tickets.

- A napkin and some train food.

- A talking tin lid with a conductor's voice asking for tickets, or with the sound of the train on the rails.

- A suitcase, or a luggage tag (as a suitcase could be a little heavy to hang!).

A trip to the beach

- bucket and spade

- sand (could use sandpaper or glue sand to the tip of the spade)

- sunscreen
- ice cream cone – the wafer could be clipped to a string even if ice cream cannot
- seaweed (if you do not live near enough to a beach to forage for your own you can make a fabric or paper representation and either soak in salt water to create a seaside smell or clip up with seaweed sheets which can be purchased from supermarkets for making sushi)
- towel
- swimwear – this could be wet to make it increase its tactile interest.

Christmas

- a spiced orange pomander
- some tinsel
- a Christmas card that plays a tune when opened
- Christmas tree edible decorations
- fairy lights (these could even be your string, so long as they were bulbs that did not glow hot).

It would be great to create a sequence that relates to a trip that the person you support is about to go on, or has recently been on. When you take a trip it is good to collect things together that you can explore later as a way of remembering or revisiting the trip through your senses.

If you work in a care setting you could consider using sensory sequences to guide people to activities; for example, if a gardening club was going to be held in the conservatory a sensory sequence could be set up along the corridor leading to the conservatory hung with items relevant to the activities that will be taking place. Think of how we might lead someone from their room to an activity, chatting to them as we go 'Come take my arm, we are going to go to the conservatory, it is time for the gardening club, you will be wanting to plant some herbs for sure' – the sensory sequence is the sensory equivalent to this gentle orientating chat. In the second case study in Section 5 Coralie shares how she uses a sensory story (itself a form of sensory sequence) to ready members of a gardening group for the activities they were to share.

A sensory topic starter

As an alternative to the more structured sensory sequence above you may like to consider compiling some sensory conversation starters around particular topics. These will be collections of items with particular sensory appeal themed around a chosen subject. You can choose to keep these items in a container of some sort or to display them, there are advantages to both options: Keeping these items in boxes or bags adds the discovery/reveal element to your conversation, whilst displaying them in some way allows people to begin the conversation at a point of their choosing and be led to a new topic within it by the choice of stimulus on offer. A conversation from a container may be led by the revealing first of one object and then another, whereas a conversation generated from a displayed collection of resources is more likely to be led by the converser's own train of thought.

As with the sensory discovery option if you are keeping items in a container of some description it is good to spend some time finding a good one, i.e. one that has particular sensory properties itself or is representative of the items within the conversation – examples could include: picnic hampers, luggage, wash bags, handbags, cardboard boxes, gift boxes, drawers, plant pots, peg bags, hat boxes and treasure chests.

If you are going to display your topic starter items then consider different ways of doing this. Choose a background against which it will be easy for a person to pick out items using their senses of touch and vision. Using a cloth or board to define the area the items are displayed in will support people in locating the items in their conversation. Present items on a slight slope so that it is easier for your conversationalist to see all of them and to reach them. Smaller items can be displayed inside a clear bowl, and it can be enjoyable to fish inside for topics of conversation. Many shops now sell clear plastic cocktail bowls which are great for this (as well as for cocktails). Another super way to display a topic of sensory conversation is to use a clothes airer meant for smalls – these hang from a single hook and have a set of pegs fixed onto them which you can use to clip sensory items to. The benefit to a hanging conversation is that it is easier to move it to be within a person's eye line, and it can be held in reach of a person wherever they happen to be. They are also easy to store as they can be hung from a rail or line.

Summary: sensory conversations

When considering what sort of sensory experience is best suited to a sensory conversation we need to take into account the impact of that experience upon the sensory system it is intended to target, i.e. will it draw the attention of that system, will it fill the perception of that sense? We also need to consider how we present it and take into account background stimuli that might mar our presentation of the experience. Understanding where the experience comes in the development of a sense can help us to choose experiences that are particularly calming or particularly likely to engage a person, with sensory experiences from early development being both calming and easiest for the brain to process.

Subtle differences in the ways in which we present experiences, from simply sharing them directly, to revealing them, or sequencing them can add dimensions of interest to sensory conversations. Sensory stories, which are addressed in the next section of this book, are a wonderful example of how developing sequences into stories unleashes a world of potential into our sensory conversation.

Section 5

Sensory stories

Orientation

Sensory stories are concise texts that partner words with sensory experiences enabling them to be accessed through our processing of language or our processing of sensory information or a combination of the two. This section gives you insight into what sensory stories are, some of the benefits they hold and advice on how to create and share your own story. In the latter half of this section you will find an example of a sensory story together with a guidance for facilitating it and suggestions for activities to accompany the story.

Sensory stories

Sensory stories are concise texts, typically less than ten sentences, in which each line of text is partnered with a richly stimulating and relevant sensory experience.

Sharing stories is a fundamental part of being human. The word 'stories' tends to first bring to mind children's books, but stories are not a thing reserved for childhood – they permeate our experience of life and to be left out from them is very alienating. Professor Penny Lacey (2006) held that sensory stories *are* literacy for those who experience meaning in a sensory way. A sensory story is not a substitute for a story; it is a story in its own right

We watch stories on the television, we read them in books and in newspapers, we use them to create and maintain our friendships. When we meet a person we share a set of stories about ourselves; this is how we introduce and explain ourselves to others. As a friendship progresses we continue to share stories to keep that bond current. To lose the ability to be able to share stories and anecdotes about oneself is to lose your ability to create and maintain relationships. Losing our linguistic abilities should not mean we have to lose this skill as well.

In Section 5 you will find a sensory story you could share with an individual with dementia, but it is my hope that as you read this book you will be motivated to create your own stories – perhaps these could be sensory stories about the person you are supporting. Do you know any of the anecdotes they used to tell, or can you find a sensory way of sharing these stories anew? Sheil (2016) concluded her research into sensory stories by surmising that they help promote the inclusion of individuals with profound disabilities by furnishing them with the opportunity to experience their environment as their peers might and to experience one-to-one communication and group communication. She notes that access to these things not only helps the individual to be included in the goings on around them but also helps them *feel* included. The difference in terms of mental health and wellbeing between feeling included and feeling alienated is huge. By creating our own sensory stories we can facilitate the inclusion of those we care for in the life around them. McKeown *et al.* (2015) report on the success of life story work for people with dementia, citing that it can improve care, offer families support, enable reflection on services and allow the voice of the person with dementia to be heard. By making life stories sensory we potentially open up these benefits to more people. Leighton *et al.*'s (2016) small-scale study suggests that this is a plausible hope.

Stories are also wonderfully supportive of memory because they hold information together in an ordered fashion. If you have ever listened to a speech or a lecture on a complicated topic in which the presenter told a story it is very likely that it is that story which your mind goes back to when you think about what they were saying. Perhaps you understood all that they said, but it is the exemplar story which they shared that anchors that information in your memory.

In this next section I am going to provide you with an overview of how to create a sensory story. For more detailed information about the benefits of sensory stories and how to create them please see: *Sensory Stories for Children and Teens* (Grace 2014). The content of the book will be relevant to anyone wishing the share sensory stories and the five stories within it are relevant to audiences of any age depending on their interests. The book also contains information about:

- using sensory stories as the basis of a group session in a variety of ways for example to calm, or to build memories

- recording ideas to support you in evaluating your sensory story sharing and building stories of greater value to your story experiencers.

Concise text

A sensory story needs concise text. The guidance I typically give is to write a story in less than ten sentences.[1] This can seem like an enormous restriction but actually reducing the language content of a story has many benefits. People worry that they will not be able to say much in so few sentences but actually it is possible to convey a lot of meaning in just a few words; the story in Section 5 is one example, and poets offer us many more. In a study (Preece and Zhao 2014) evaluating the incredibly popular sensory stories produced by the charity Bag Books among the few negative criticisms received were comments that some stories were too long and complicated or were not personal enough. In creating your own text you can create both a personalised and concise text which will be a wonderful resource to share.

All of our brains have a limited processing capacity and when we are struggling with our health, be that mental or physical, our resources are depleted. Language places huge processing demands on the brain. You will know from times when you have felt stressed

---

1 This is in line with guidance given by other organisations that create and share sensory stories, for example PAMIS and Bag Books.

or ill that you need peace and quiet, you do NOT want lots and lots of words. By reducing the number of words we use in a conversation, or whilst sharing a story, we reduce the demands we place on someone's processing capacity and thus we make it easier for them to listen to us.

We take in more information when less is said; politicians know this and use it to their advantage by providing us with soundbites rather than speeches. Although a well-reasoned speech clearly contains more information than a succinct soundbite we remember more information from the soundbite than we do from the speech. A story distilled to its essence and shared in a few words will go deeper into us than a long and rambling tale.

Options

- Retreating text, building text, concise text: In your use of concise text as you create a sensory story to share with someone with dementia you may want to consider the following story options:

- Concise text: Create a concise story of just a few sentences (between 6 and 10); share the story using only these sentences and allowing plenty of time to explore the meaning conveyed through the accompanying experiences.

- Retreating text: Create a concise text version of a pre-existing longer story. This is ideal for if you are creating a sensory story about an event in a person's life that they currently remember in part. This is the approach that myself and my co-authors of Dementia Life stories (Leighton *et al.* 2016) used when creating a life story for an individual with dementia.

A good way to do this is to write out the story in full and then look for the sentences that make its backbone, the essence of the narrative, then use these as paragraph headings. So for example a paragraph heading might be 'They got married' and the content of that paragraph would be a more detailed explanation of the wedding.

When you share a retreating text story you use as much language as the person you are sharing the story with is able to enjoy. So perhaps when you begin telling the story you are sharing it in full, but later on, when the journey into dementia has progressed you may just be sharing the paragraph headings and a few bits and pieces of detail and eventually it will just be the paragraph headings that are shared. Be careful to reduce the language promptly when needed, if you continue to share the story with more language than the person can process it will become an alienating experience for them and not the shared conversational experience you intend. If in doubt always use less language not more.

It is important that when sharing a retreating text story you plan from the start what the bare bones of the story will be and always share these sentences in the same way, using the same turn of phrase each time so that the person hearing the story hears these particular sentences repeated over and over again, associated with the broader content of the story. This will give them the maximum chance of connecting with their meaning as their journey into dementia progresses.

- Building text: Create a concise story of between 6 and 10 sentences that you feel are likely to resonate with the person with whom you are sharing the story. You will then share the story and allow space for them to build on its content with their own insights, recollections, ideas and opinions.

Coralie's example in the second case study in Section 5 is a building text sensory story.

It is most likely that if you are creating a building text story, you will look to create a story that brings back old memories. If you are doing this, choosing story content that relates to the late teens or early twenties of the person with whom you are sharing the story is likely to be most fruitful. However connection with memory is not the only route to a building text story. It can be nice to consider other options so that we avoid constantly asking people to access their memory banks. Other options are to create a fantasy story or a comment story:

- Fantasy story creation can be a fun shared activity with younger family members – perhaps the person with dementia can help to tell a story to the children about unicorns and dragons and other such creatures.

- A comment story would be one about a topic on which the person hearing the story is likely to have opinions. The word 'story' suggests narrative, but we can stretch that a bit to include short commentaries; for example, a few sentences on motor car racing, or gardening, or the problem with pigeons in the square.

As you share a building text story you will share the concise text of the story and leave space for the person you are sharing it with to build upon that with their own comments, observations, suggestions or opinions.

Rich and relevant stimuli

Each sentence of your story is going to be partnered with a rich and relevant sensory experience. Meaning will be expressed through these experiences. The sensory experiences within a sensory story are just as important as the words of the story and should be held in equal regard.

Ideally over the course of the story you will be offering stimulation to a wide range of sensory systems.

Getting your choice of experience right is very rewarding as well-chosen experiences generate greater engagement with the story, hold people's concentration, stimulate their thoughts and ideas, and foster connection between you as the storyteller and them as the story experiencer.

In the next section we are going to spend a bit of time looking at what makes a really great sensory experience for a sensory story, or indeed for any sensory conversation you are planning.

Repeat

Once you have a super sensory story created with concise text and rich and relevant sensory experiences you are going to look to share it with the person for whom it was created a great many times. Told consistently over time sensory stories can be used to develop emergent communication skills and foster engagement with the world (Penne *et al.* 2012; Ten Brug *et al.* 2012; PAMIS 2002; Taylor 2006 in Grace and Silva 2017). In an ideal world of sensory story sharing the same person would facilitate the sensory story each time. It is unlikely that, unless you are the primary carer yourself and plan to always be the one to share the story, this is possible. A good second best is to arrange for a small group of people to take responsibility for sharing the sensory story and for this small group to work collaboratively to try and ensure consistency between how each person shares the story.

If possible, aim to be the person that tells the story repeatedly, or for the story to be told consistently by a select group of people. Grace and Silvia (2017) found that the prime storyteller was a critical component in the increased responsiveness of participants over time during sensory story telling. Grace and Silvia also found that sharing sensory stories enhanced social interactions and strengthened the bonds between the participants and the storyteller.

Repetition is a strategy most of us turn to when looking to support our own memory. If someone asks you to remember a sequence of numbers for them most probably you repeat them aloud until they ask you for them. In repeating a sensory story we are hoping to foster memory in this way, but this is not the only reason for the repetition.

By repeating a story we create a situation, both in language and sensory experience, that is predictable and familiar to the person who has experienced the repetition. When an experience is predictable and feels familiar we feel safe within that experience. And when we feel safe we are better able to take in information and engage. So although it can seem like we are saying something we have said before and nothing new can be gained from doing that, in repeating a sensory story we may actually be offering someone something new each time as each time they hear and experience it, so they are able to access and take in a little more of it. Typically story experiencers show an increase in responses after repeated telling rather than a drop off[2] (Grace and Silvia 2017; Leighton *et al.* 2016; Ten Brug *et al.* 2012; Lambe and Hogg 2013; PAMIS 2002; Taylor 2006; Watson 2002; Young *et al.* 2011; Young and Lambe 2011). People do not get bored – their interest grows and they become more engaged. It is almost certain that you, as the facilitator of the story, will get bored long before the repeating of the story becomes meaningless. One of the great skills in facilitating a sensory story is not the maintaining of interest from your audience but the maintaining of your own interest and engagement with the story. As the storyteller you need to be involved in the narrative yourself, no one is interested in a story whose teller is bored.

Sharing a sensory story

Here are five tips for sharing a sensory story, taken from refining the guidance for sensory story telling by Grace and Silva (2017).

1. Facilitators should read the story text and share the related experience clearly, aiming to do this in the same way each time they share the story

Repetition of experience supports a person in understanding what is going on. For example, if you were to navigate to a new place you would at first need a lot of support to guide you there but after a few attempts it would become familiar to you. You would be able

---

2   Much of the research into the benefits of repeated sensory story telling is carried out on the population of people with profound disabilities, not the population of people with dementia (with a few exceptions). Whilst there are clear differences between these groups it seems reasonable to believe that findings for the first group would be similarly reflected in the second group. Both groups access the stories in spite of severe intellectual and physical challenges to doing so. Studies that have looked at sensory stories as an intervention for people with dementia support this belief, for example: Leighton *et al.* (2016).

to find your way based on the familiar sights and sounds around you. In a sensory story a person's understanding is supported by keeping everything the same. Your navigation would not be improved by going a different route each time. Likewise a sensory story is not improved by having it varied.

Sometimes people reading the stories can feel that it is boring to read them in the same way each time, or that it is of little significance if a bell rung as a sound experience is red on one telling and blue on another. We need to remember that the consistency of experience is not for us, it is for the person with whom we are sharing the story, and whilst small changes might not seem like a big deal to us they can be critical to the person experiencing the story. It can seem simple to repeat, but this assumption of simplicity fosters a carelessness to the repetition and the impact of the stories is lessened. A research team working in the Netherlands and Belgium, Ten Brug *et al.* (2012), looked at how sensory stories were shared across 29 activity centres and found that even under research conditions tellers found it difficult to maintain consistency in their story telling. So whilst the instruction to repeat the story in the same way can sound simple we know it is actually quite a challenge – but a challenge worth meeting.

Think of your navigation through that unfamiliar environment; perhaps you remember that it is a left turn at the blue door. Maybe if I were to navigate that same route I would not even notice the blue door, I would just know to walk towards the sound of the music pouring out of the music shop on the left-hand side. If you were to walk the route and find someone had painted the blue door red you might get lost. We use the details of our world to understand where we are. Someone experiencing a sensory story will use the details of that experience to hang their understanding onto. Even the slightest change can leave someone lost.

By thinking about how we will phrase the story ahead of time, where we will pause, where we will add drama to our voice, we can ensure that we say the words of the story in the same way each time. Similarly by thinking about how we will facilitate the sensory experiences, for example if there is a bell to ring will we ring it just once or will we clang it back and forth for a while, we can ensure the same predictability of experience. If you are sharing a sensory story that builds text or a sensory story that is reducing in text try to keep the backbone of the story, that core which is the few sentences and the experiences, the same each time even if that which is around it varies.

2. Facilitators should allow time for reactions and responses

When we share a story we are engaged in a communicative act, and all communication is turn taking in nature. You may not receive responses in the same way as you communicate the story; that is to say you will not necessarily receive words in exchange for your words or engagement with a stimulus in exchange for an experience but more than likely there will be a response there.

Allow time for that response; show recognition of it. Your recognition does not have to be verbal, the best kind would be that delivered through the same medium as the response. So if the response was someone leaning in to you, you could lean in to them. If the response was a sound you could join in with that sound, and so on.

The word 'time' is important in this piece of advice. We are used to receiving responses very promptly, indeed we often communicate with people who begin to respond before we have even finished what we are saying. As people's processing time gets slower there will be a delay before a response is produced. If you always begin your next part in the communication before time is allowed for a response it is as if you are having a conversation with someone but constantly cutting off what they were going to say next. It is very likely that if you did that your conversation partner would quickly lose interest in talking to you. Processing time can vary enormously and can be different on different days; if someone is feeling ill or has not slept much, the time it takes them to be respond can be longer than usual. For some people a response will take several minutes to formulate. It can be hard to sit and hold space with a person as you wait for a response that takes minutes to come, but what a wonderful thing to be able to do: to be the person who hears a person who is normally unheard. What a precious role to play in someone's life, to be the one who waits long enough to hear them.

3. Facilitators should refrain from adding extra language to the story in order to keep the experience of the story consistent and allow the experiencer to focus on the experiences

Language places a heavy burden on the processing centres in our brains. For those of us used to indulging in language day in, day out it is less noticeable, although the effect is still there. For people struggling with language it is much more noticeable. It can be very easy to add words to a sensory story, especially when facilitating the experiences. For some people these words will be a companionable part of the experience and they are absolutely fine. But for other people these words will place a burden on their processing that blocks out their opportunity to fully experience the sensory stimuli offered or wears them out before the communication exchange has finished.

Typically the language added to a story has little content or meaning itself; it is often the froth of our language, the small talk, niceties and pleasantries that we use to fill the gaps. We find this sort of verbiage reassuring because language reassures us. But language to a person struggling to process language can be distressing. Imagine yourself in a foreign country where you only know a few words of the language spoken. Would you prefer a companion who speaks the mother tongue of the country to babble at you constantly, or would you be grateful if they stuck to just the few words you could understand and said these in a clear uncluttered fashion? If a person is not outputting language they do not need you to output enough for two – they need you to feel comfortable being with them in their silence. It takes a bit of practice but you can do it, and you may find you enjoy the new subtleties of this type of communication.

4. Ideally facilitators should know the person they are sharing the story with and be aware of their sensory abilities and preferences

It would be wonderful if every person who shared a sensory story with another knew that other person really well. Knew what they were likely to enjoy, what might worry them, knew whether their hearing was perfect or whether it was fading, their vision 20:20 or long sighted or short sighted. Clearly this sort of facilitation is often the stuff of dreams. A study by Vlaskamp *et al.* (2007) found care staff had little knowledge of the sensory abilities and preferences of the people in their care and were liable to interpret their reactions to stimuli through their own experience rather than attempting to perceive the world as experienced by the individual being cared for. You may be a practitioner supporting individuals with dementia in a big residential care setting. You know your clients well but you do not have mountains of knowledge on each one – you have to simply do your best. But as you do your best try to notice where you get engagement and where you do not. Build up a mental picture of each person's sensory preferences and use this to inform what you do as you share further stories in the future. If you would like further support in doing this, the 'Getting to know you questions' in Grace (2014, Part IV 10b) are based on Vlaskamp *et al.*'s research and intended to give you an awareness of what you need to find out.

5. Facilitators need to prepare for sharing a sensory story thoroughly, ensuring all resources are ready for use before the story begins

This one sounds so simple – but as simple as it is to say, so simple is it to get wrong. Because you are looking to facilitate the same experiences with a sensory story in the same way each time the best thing you can do is to collect the resources you need for a particular story together and then keep them in a box or bag so that they are always to hand ready for the story to be shared. If you have to go and find them each time you are likely to get slightly different things or lose an item.

Check things like batteries before you begin a story. If you plan to use a torch or a small sound-making device it is no good discovering its batteries are flat when you are halfway through the story. Get into the habit of making simple checks first.

Before you begin your story lay the resources you are going to use to tell it out in such a way that they will be easily accessible to you as you tell the story. Untangle things that might need untangling. Place things that will be accessed in order such that the one you will need soonest is on top. It is all obvious stuff but so very easy to get wrong. In typical spoken communication little muddles do not matter, but for those with greater needs the confusions become a barrier to engagement and understanding. If you can keep your sharing of a sensory story consistent throughout then you maximise the chances of being able to reach someone with it who would not be reached through other means. In other words the little bit of prep and fuss is completely worth it.

A common thread to all of the advice points above is the desire to keep things consistent. The idea that repetition is boring is learned. Most of us when we first encountered stories wanted to hear our favourite ones over and over again. Many of us turn to well-known stories in books or films for comfort in times of need. We love telling stories that relate to ourselves and relish the opportunity to tell them again and connect with good times.

Once you discover the power of consistently sharing sensory stories you may seek to increase the continuity of experience, perhaps by always sharing the story in the same location, or at the same time of day. How often you repeat a story is also significant. For some people a weekly story may be enough to keep them in touch with it; other people will benefit from hearing a story daily.

Case studies: sensory dementia

Examples from Coralie Oddy at Reminisense. Notice that in Case Study 2 Coralie is using a building text model of a sensory story.

Case study 1 – the hat box

With a special 85th birthday celebration coming up for Doreen Graham, a woman with vascular dementia as the result of a stroke, a lovely opportunity for sensory exploration presented itself. Doreen's daughter Laura had organised a Mad Hatter's tea party, so that Doreen's carers and loved ones could drop by – in some eye catching hats – to chat and share some of Doreen's favourite food and music, without overwhelming her with too many guests at once.

I prepared a sensory box of hat decorations for Doreen and I to explore together in advance of her party. As well as providing a basis for interaction – a conversation that would be built through joint exploration and discovery – the sensory box was also designed to prepare Doreen for her party. By creating an object together (in this case, a decorated hat) I hoped to build a sense of familiarity around the event in which the object would be used.

I put the hat decorations into a brown shoebox, tied loosely with some parcel string. Visually, this conjured reminiscence of a newly arrived parcel – an exciting package to open with eager hands – and I treated it as such to capture Doreen's interest in the box and its contents. I built anticipation by drumming my fingertips against the box, wondering aloud 'What's inside?' Doreen was sometimes anxious about exploring objects with her hands and tended to put them down quickly, but the rough parcel string seemed a comforting texture to rub between her finger and thumb. Doreen's slight tugging of the string relaxed and loosened it, providing a natural opportunity to open the box.

Because of Doreen's reluctance to handle objects and limited vision, I supported her to explore the objects by holding each one in her eye line and offering it towards her. Doreen would show interest in an object by inclining her head towards it and narrowing her eyes, sometimes commenting on what she saw. Other objects she would dismiss or look past. In this way she made choices about which objects to explore further.

I chose each object for its potential to be explored in a variety of ways. A scrap of patterned chiffon could be scented with a spray of perfume and smelt, drawn gently across Doreen's forearm to provide a cool, tickling sensation, or held up at eye height and looked through, casting the whole room in colourful patterns. A string of beads would catch the light and sparkle when gently swung, and also produce a pleasing clattering sound when rubbed between the hands. A colourful fan created a new pattern when moved rapidly, and wafted a cool breeze onto Doreen's face.

Doreen responded to these sensory experiences in different ways. Invited to smell, she would inhale deeply and often comment on the scents presented to her. For her, a scent seemed to provide a powerful connection with the present moment and gave her opportunities to raise her own reflections and opinions, often through speech but also through facial expressions and physically seeking out the scent again. Scenting objects for Doreen sometimes created a 'hook' to draw her into further engagement with the object through her other senses. Once intrigued by the smell, the colour or sound of the object sometimes became more salient or meaningful to her too.

While Doreen gave clear responses to sights and smells, her reactions to touch and sound were often more subtle; for example, a slight stiffening or change in breathing. It was important to give her time to process each sensation and respond in her own way.

If an object was pleasing to Doreen, I would suggest attaching it to one of the hats for the Mad Hatter's tea party – a dark hat to provide a strong visual contrast to the hat decorations, with a wide brim to bear their weight. Each time we attached a new item, we used Doreen's mirror to admire how the hat looked on her, building her familiarity with wearing it. As we did this, Doreen would often look intently into the mirror, and suddenly break into a dazzling smile. She could see her reflection in a costume which was novel and surprising, but also full of personal familiarity thanks to her unique sensory engagement with each of the hat's decorations – and she liked what she saw.

Case study 2 – going dancing

With limited vision and mobility, Doreen liked to sit with her family and carers listening to music, sometimes singing along to familiar tunes. Because she was so responsive to music – and a regular at the dance hall during her youth – I decided to share a sensory story about a couple who meet at a dance in the 1950s with Doreen.

I had shared this story ('Going Dancing', ReminiSense) before with a group at a dementia-friendly tea dance. Normally I would say each line of the story and move around the circle, sharing each new sensory experience with each person in turn, until the story was completed. At the end of the story I would encourage reflections and give opportunities to explore the sensory objects again. Occasionally, the people I shared the story with would alter the flow of it in their own ways – most notably by including a spontaneous group rendition of 'Singin' in the Rain' – but essentially I retained control of how the story was told. I wondered if there was a way to retain the story's structure whilst giving greater control to its listeners to shape it as they saw fit.

With Doreen, we adopted a far more open, conversational approach. Due to her fleeting attention and occasional hallucinations, as well as her ability to verbally comment, give opinions and reminisce when fully engaged, we found the story was shared most effectively by me reading the first line and sharing the sensory experience, and using this as a springboard for Doreen to add to the story. Doreen's daughter Laura sat with us and offered some great reminiscences that Doreen had passed on to her through previous conversations – these gave each line of the story a range of personal interpretations and associations for Doreen to draw on and add her own input to. For example:

- *Me:* 'It was Saturday night at the Palais…' *(I start to play Big Band music and offer a mirror ball to Doreen.)*

- *Laura:* I think you used to go out to dance on a Saturday night, with your sister.

- *Doreen:* Oh, most nights of the week.

We would allow the conversation to pass back and forth in a natural away until Doreen lost focus – at this point Laura and I would wonder aloud what would happen next in the story, and give the next line and sensory experience. This helped to refocus Doreen and draw her gently back into reminiscing with us without putting her under any pressure. In this way we were able to keep the conversation flowing for an hour without having to ask Doreen direct questions or give any explicit reminders of what we were talking about, which could have increased her anxiety by drawing attention to her memory difficulties – something Doreen was very aware of and commented on frequently.

In contrast, handling tap shoes and being supported to tap and clatter them on the table top allowed her to reminisce about taking her daughter to dance classes. The scent of Brylcreem led to memories of how she met her husband and the dances he attended with her, whilst listening to 'Singin' in the Rain' supported recollections of how Grace Kelly became a princess.

Rather than feeling I was telling a story, I felt all three of us were fully involved in the story's form and creation – and it was a richer experience for all of us because of that.

Laura reported that for weeks after this reminiscence session, she and Doreen would regularly reminisce about the session and content, as follows:

- *Laura*: Mum, I remember when Coralie came and you were telling us about when you used to go dancing with your sister.

- *Doreen*: Yes, I remember, we had the music on.

- *Laura*: Shall I put the music on now, and you tell me all about your dancing days?

- *Doreen*: Oh, that would be nice.

Sensory story

Here is a sensory story for you to share with an individual with dementia. If you choose to share it I hope you get a lot of pleasure from doing so, but more than that I hope you will be inspired to create your own personalised stories as these will be far more powerful than anything I can create.

Suggested story topics

- Create a sensory story inspired by a tale you know the person you are supporting loves (e.g. the witches mixing their potion in Shakespeare's *Macbeth*).

- Create a sensory story based on a trip you plan on taking. The benefit to a story like this is you can use it ahead of your outing to prepare the person you are supporting for the experiences they will encounter.

- Create a sensory story out of a familiar family anecdote and use actual items from the event in the story to convey the sensory narrative.

- Create a sensory story about yourself.

- Create a sensory story about an event in history you think will be of interest to the person you are supporting.

- Create a sensory story about a current event or a current television series.

- Create a sensory story about a care routine – sharing the story can help the person you support to understand the care sequence.

- Create a sensory story about an activity that you shared together (e.g. a day trip you shared or a craft activity you took part in together).

- Create a sensory story based on a significant life event (e.g. the birth of a child).

- Create a sensory story that focuses on taking care of a pet.

- Create a sensory story about a particular culture or country.

- Create a sensory story about a friend of the person whom you are supporting.

- Create a sensory story based around a favourite hobby or interest (e.g. a story about gardening).

A sensory story with supporting activity ideas

Below you will find the text to the sensory story 'The Gardener's New Grandchild', along with brief prompts that relate to the sensory experiences intended to accompany the text. After the story you will find a more detailed explanation of each of the experiences along with tips about how to resource and facilitate them. I will also explain some of the choices I made when writing the story as these may help you when you create your own stories. Once you've read this section you will be able to share the story using just the text below.

The gardener's new grandchild

Neighbours hear the footsteps of the old gardener as he walks down the hill to his garden.

Patting hands, as if footsteps.

They smile at one another as he passes and whisper, 'He must have had the news.'

Smiles and whispers.

The gardener's fingers toy with an acorn in his pocket; it is hard and round and smooth beneath his touch.

Hold an acorn or wooden bead.

The gardener whistles happily to himself as he opens the garden gate and steps inside.

Happy whistling, a familiar tune, possibly a gate's squeak.

He pauses for a moment to take a long slow breath of the heady air. Flowers grow all around and their fragrance is everywhere.

Floral scent.

The gardener walks over to the old oak tree, grown from an acorn planted on the day that he was born, and rests his hand on its rough bark.

Feel the texture of bark.

The leaves of the great tree shelter the gardener from the sun and whisper their congratulations gently as they rustle in the wind.

Shade and leaves rustling.

After a while the gardener steps out of the shade of the tree and walks to an open patch of earth.

Shade/light/soil tray.

He kneels and digs a hole with his hands, then he takes the acorn from his pocket and pushes it deep into the hold before covering it with soil and patting it down tenderly. 'Grow well', he whispers.

Plant seed in soil.

The gardener's new grandchild – explanation of story and resources

Neighbours hear the footsteps of the old gardener as he walks down the hill to his garden.

The story starts gently – we are hoping to draw people in with an experience they can be a part of and gradually gain more attention and interest as the story progresses until at the end of the story we hope they will take part in the activity of planting the seed with as much independence as is appropriate to the individual.

To create the auditory and proprioceptive experience of the gardener's footsteps we are going to use the flats of our hands to pat out the sound of his footsteps against our thighs or against a table top.

You may be sharing this story one to one, in which case you could pat your own legs with a footstep rhythm and encourage the person you are sharing the story with to copy you, or you could begin by patting your own legs and then move across to pat theirs and then move back again, to give the impression of the gardener walking at first closer to them and then further away as he passes them on his way to his garden.

If you are sharing this story with a group of people it can be fun to begin the footstep sound yourself by sitting in front of the group and demonstrating clearly the rhythmic pat, pat, pat against your thighs, but then move around the circle patting each person in turn, or patting the table in front of them, as if you are the gardener and they are the neighbours you are passing. You can encourage people to join in the patting; perhaps more and more people will join in as you move around the circle so that the sound stimulus builds; perhaps people will join in as you reach them but then stop after you have passed, creating the effect of the gardener's footsteps passing by.

A gentle building rhythm is a wonderful way to get people involved. Beats are naturally joined in with – if you keep this beat quite steady and slow, like a strong heartbeat it will be reassuring as well as involving. The opportunity for connection through touch is another important way of inviting people to participate and connecting with them in a non-verbal way. Another option not explored for the patting above is to have it travel over a person's body – you could pat the gardener's footsteps up one of their arms, across their shoulders, and down their other arm, as if they were a hill the gardener had walked over. Patting the body is great for promoting an awareness of where the body is in space and so is a lovely supportive stimulus for proprioception.

This slow steady gentle start to the story should awaken people's interest without distressing them and invite them to walk with the gardener.

If you wanted to set the various parts of the story out around a room or outside space at different stations then story sharers could actually walk with the gardener through the story, which would be wonderful.

Before you choose how to facilitate these stimuli think about who you will be sharing the story with, where you will be when you share the story for the first time and also where you are likely to be for future tellings of the story. Remember you are aiming to tell the story in the same way each time.

If it suits your story experiencer/experiencers you can continue the sound of the footsteps through the next sentence of the story as well.

They smile at one another as he passes and whisper, 'He must have had the news.'

Take this sentence slowly, make time for the smile to be there on its own, perhaps pausing after the word smile to smile as broadly and as gladly as you can. For these neighbours to know why the gardener is passing they must be old friends. Maybe the gardener lives in a little village with people he has known his whole life – he will have been chatting to them in the shops telling them his daughter is pregnant, and he has told the whole town that the baby is due any day now, so when they see him from their windows, from the bus stop, from the shop, walking with purpose to his garden at the bottom of the village, they know why and they are deeply glad for him. These words, of course, are not in the story, the feeling of these words is what your smile must convey.

Once you have shared your warm smile the whispering of 'He must have heard the news' is the beginning of the drama of the story. These are the words that invite you to get involved in this man's life. As you whisper them summon up all your acting skills and fill your whisper with intrigue.

If you are sharing the story one to one you will smile and whisper directly at the person with whom you are sharing the story. If you are sharing the story in a group it is good to make sure everyone has been smiled at, if possible one to one. The whisper can be delivered to the whole group at once – you will need a few more acting skills to do this as you seek to do an 'on stage' whisper, projecting it so everyone can hear it. Alternatively you could walk amongst the group and whisper into people's ears as if passing on gossip – done with a glint of mischief in the eye this can be quite fun and can wrap everyone up in a spirited community atmosphere.

Smiling in response to someone else smiling is very natural. We have mirror neurons in our brains that are dedicated to copying the emotional responses we see in others. Our mirror neurons help us to empathise as when we see emotion they enable us to feel a little of it too. Smiling releases hormones in the brain that make us feel happy. So although we may smile when we feel happy, we also feel happy when we smile, making smiling a good form of therapy. If you can smile so deeply and sincerely that you generate smiles in your story experiencers then, not only do you give them the warmth of your smile you also create a piece of happiness within them. Which is why taking time and putting everything into the smile is absolutely worth it.

If you are sharing the story one to one you probably already have a good awareness of what your story experiencer's vision is like and so are well placed to position your smile somewhere where they will clearly see it. If you are working in a group it is possible that you will be sharing the story with people you are not so familiar with. A 'best bet' for facilitating a visual experience is to position it in front of someone's face, in their direct line of sight taking into account where their eyes are looking as you present the stimulus; so if someone is looking down you would position the stimulus low down, likewise if someone was looking up you might raise the stimulus up. When not engaged most people's eyesight rests at a distance that is about elbow length away from their face (their own elbow) so it can be useful to hold stimuli at about this distance from them in order to generate engagement. In terms of facilitating a smile as a visual experience this means you will need to move your head so that it is facing theirs, meet their eyes with your own if appropriate and come closer to them than you might otherwise. Of course as you do this you will be noticing their responses and judging whether they are positive or negative and adjusting what you do accordingly.

> The gardener's fingers toy with an acorn in his pocket, it is
> hard and round and smooth beneath his touch.

Depending on whether your story experiencer participated in the patting footsteps at the start of this story or not it is possible for a story experiencer to have reached this line of the story having been a passive recipient of the story. This is the first line where we are looking for active participation.

The experience is going to be a tactile one of touching the acorn or wooden bead representing the acorn. Presenting the acorn or bead within a pocket of some sort is a great way to add a little sensory curiosity to the telling of the story. You can use a simple fabric pouch, or the pocket of an actual coat. You can demonstrate the presence of the acorn by reaching into the pocket yourself, taking it out and playing with it in your fingers as you read this line, before offering the pocket with the acorn inside to your story experiencer/experiencers to explore.

The nice thing about using a pocket for this experience is that if you are facilitating the story for someone still involved in a passive way it is possible to slip the pocket over their hand so that their fingertips brush against the acorn inside and in this way encourage interaction with the stimulus.

As with all the experiences, allow time. Allow time for the object to be touched, and processed. It may be that the roughness of an acorn's cup to the touch, or the smoothness of its surface, brings back a hint of a memory and although that memory cannot always be expressed the sensation holds it in the mind. Try to remain silent as you allow your story experiencer to touch the acorn. Your words can drown out subtle sensory memories. Trust that the story is being told by the experience.

> The gardener whistles happily to himself as he opens the
> garden gate and steps inside.

With this stimulus the story continues to build in its efforts to engage and interest. Whistling is often used to alert people and songs are very good tools for getting people to join in. If you are facilitating this experience for a story experiencer/experiencers who are likely to need a little bit of a 'wake up' then perform a loud whistle that changes pitch, a siren-like whistle. If you know a tune likely to appeal to your story's audience then whistle that. Remember as you facilitate the story for the first time that you are going to be looking to repeat the story in the same way on multiple tellings. In a care environment it may be that you are sharing the story telling with another member of staff and so will need to agree between you the tune you plan on whistling. However you are sharing the story make a note of the sort of whistle you use when you first share the story and then try to stick to that on future tellings. There may be some circumstances where you would look to change the whistle, for example, if someone is distressed by the sound you first choose, or someone joins in and whistles a tune of their own.

> He pauses for a moment to take a long slow breath of the heady air. Flowers grow all around and their fragrance is everywhere.

You can use any floral scent you wish for this stimulus. Fresh flowers would be wonderful and even if you cannot get the same ones every time you tell the story the benefits of having actual flowers are likely to outweigh the disadvantage of slightly inconsistent stimuli from one telling to the next. However, you may be keen to ensure exactly the same olfactory experience is offered on each telling of the story, or you may be concerned about allergies to pollen and so wish to use a synthetic scent.

Essential oils are cheap to purchase and offer a wide range of bold scent experiences. Typically, a bottle of essential oil is priced around one or two pounds and shops that sell them stock a great variety of scents. Taking in the advice from Section 4 you might look to choose a heavy base note floral scent such as lavender or camomile to represent the smell of the flowers in the gardener's garden or a very sweet smell like vanilia or ylangylang or even a sweet musk such as a white musk.

If you choose to use an essential oil as the stimulus for this section of the story pop a few drops of it onto a natural fibre pad or swatch of fabric (e.g. a cotton wool pad, or a swatch of cotton) and seal this inside a small plastic container. Doing this means that the air inside the container becomes fragranced making for a bolder smell experience when the lid is lifted. Prior to telling the story you will want to check that the smell is still fresh and bold when you take the lid off. If it is not then you will need to add a few new drops of oil to the cloth inside.

To facilitate the experience simply remove the lid from the container and pass it slowly beneath someone's nose. You can model the slow steady breath in that the gardener takes in the story. Discourage swift sniffing as people are less likely to pick up the scent molecules in the air that way. People are also less likely to be able to access a smell experience if they are dehydrated so ensuring everyone has had a glass of water before you begin to tell the story or has water on hand to sip when they wish is another way of supporting this experience.

As with all the experiences, take your time and try not to talk over it. Allow the meaning of the experience to be taken in with the senses and connected with, without rushing on to the next line too soon.

The gardener walks over to the oak tree, grown from an acorn planted on the day that he was born, and rests his hand on its rough bark.

The ideal resource for this experience would be a piece of bark, gnarled and rough. If you cannot find a piece of bark then you are looking for something bark-like. One option can be to make your own out of cardboard and brown tissue paper. To do this you would glue strips of cardboard onto a piece of card to emulate the rough surface of bark and then layer over with tissue paper wet with a mixture of glue and water. Left to dry the tissue paper will mould itself around the strips of cardboard to create a surface similar to the surface of a piece of bark.

Story experiencers who are able to and who are engaged in the story, as hopefully everyone will be by this point in the narrative, can reach out and rest their hand against the bark as if they are the gardener resting their hand against the tree. You can support story experiencers experiencing the story in a more passive way to engage in this experience by lifting their hand on top the bark and letting it rest there for a while.

If lifting someone's hand onto a touch experience it can feel natural to lift their hand by placing your hand over the back of their hand and lifting it. Of course this works, it gets their hand where you hoped to get it but there is more to think about than that. Flo Longhorn taught me that it can be more supportive to lift someone's hand by sliding your own underneath it and then sliding it off your hand onto the stimulus being offered. Think about the difference between these methods of facilitating touch. Someone experiencing the first one feels a touch on the back of their hands which encloses them; they then have their hand pressed against another object. To opt out of the experience they would have to assert themselves with a degree of force. The first touch experience they encounter during the facilitation is to the back of their hand, drawing their attention to the back of their hand when actually we want their attention to be on the more sensitive underside of their hand which we are going to present to the stimulus.

Using the underneath the hand slide approach to facilitating a touch experience means that the first sensations of the experience are to the sensitive underside of the hand, readying it for the experience about to be presented. If your hand is balanced on top of someone else's hand it is relatively easy to pull away. The subtlety of this method of facilitating touch not only provides a way of moving someone's hand from one location to another but allows for agency within the experience which is so important for respecting an individual and preserving their self-esteem.

Sometimes people think that when someone appears to be entirely passive or unresponsive during a sensory story, there is little point in sharing the story with them. This is a very sad misunderstanding. These seemingly unresponsive people are often those for whom the sensory world is the most important. Allowing them extra time with an experience can begin to reveal their connection, and if you give them extended time to absorb an experience you may see a flicker of recognition or get a tiny response. To be providing the experience that reaches them when nothing else is getting through is very, very precious. Even without seeing that flicker of recognition or tiny motion of response it is worth offering and allowing time for these experiences. You cannot know what is happening inside of them. It might be that the touch of that bark against their skin brings to mind the wisp of a memory of a time when they leant upon a tree, perhaps stopping on a country walk to admire the view, or leaning back against a tree to be kissed by their lover whilst courting. Give them the time. Give them the experience. The skill of facilitation when supporting someone who seems entirely passive is often the skill of holding yourself in that moment, without getting bored, without filling with language, without fidgeting, just being happy to be in that moment together. This can take practice but it will be good for you as well as for them.

> The leaves of the great tree shelter the gardener from the sun and whisper their congratulations gently as they rustle in the wind.

The sibilant sound of leaves rustling is a lovely soothing white noise sound. Creating this noise is another great chance for involvement in the creation of the sensory side of this narrative. The easiest way to create the stimulus is to use a tree branch with leaves on and shake it as the wind would. If you can have enough branches so that everyone experiencing the story has one to hold you can all work together to create this sound stimulus.

Of course not everyone has trees growing outside their place which they can snap branches off at will so it is necessary to look for an alternative way to create this sound. We have lots of options. It is relatively easy to access sound clips online via sites like YouTube or SoundCloud, in this way you can play your story experiencer/experiencers the sound of leaves. But this option does not allow for the group participation that having branches does. Paper rustling makes the right sort of noise. It is simple to make paper branches and provide these for people to rustle. You can make these out of plain paper or you can use tree colours, browns and greens, to create something that more visually represents the stimulus we are aiming at.

To make a paper tree branch you need two pieces of paper, one brown, one green. Roll the brown sheet of paper along the long edge and use two pieces of sellotape to secure the roll, placing one piece at the bottom of the roll and one piece slightly below the middle. Take a pair of scissors and insert them into the top of the roll; cut down to the middle of the roll (so just before you reach the middle piece of sellotape), and make several cuts like this so that the top of the roll is now frayed by your cuts. Pinch the inside fronds of cut paper and pull them gently upwards – they will untwist slightly as you pull them upwards and the paper fronds will hang down all around. Now cut leaf shapes out of the green piece of paper and glue these to the ends of the brown fronds. Once the glue is dry you have a tree branch that is easy to hold onto and when waved will make a soft rustling sound like the leaves of a tree swaying in the wind.

Once again take the time to allow the sound of this experience to be appreciated and absorbed, respecting that the sound itself maybe conveying more meaning to your story experiencer(s) than the words you speak as you tell the story.

> After a while the gardener steps out of the shade of the tree and walks to an open patch of earth.

This is a very gentle experience and is essentially a preparation for the final experience of the story where we are hoping for maximum engagement from our story experiencers. If you wish to make it a visual experience you can emphasise the light and shade using the leaf branches from the preceding sentence to create shade and drawing them back to allow for light. You can even support this by turning lights off and then switching them on. However what we are hoping to do is begin to focus attention on the soil into which we will plant our acorns or wooden beads or whatever has been used to represent the acorn in the story.

I would suggest having a small box or tray of earth for each story experiencer. These can be purchased at little expense from garden centres or online but more often than not fruit and veg is sold in plastic packaging that would be perfect for this experience: relatively deep and transparent. In an ideal world you want a tray that is deep enough to allow your story experiencer to dig a little in the soil with their fingers and bury something beneath it. If the tray is also transparent that is a bonus as it means the soil can be clearly seen from all angles. If you are not using a transparent tray try to choose one that is muted in tone as a brightly coloured or decorated one can detract attention from the soil which is to be the focus of the upcoming experience.

The tray of soil can be presented through the facilitation of this experience by holding the branches of leaves over it and then withdrawing them to reveal it as you talk about the gardener in the story walking to the open patch of earth.

> He kneels and digs a hole with his hands, then he takes the acorn from his pocket and pushes it deep into the hold before covering it with soil and patting it down tenderly. 'Grow well', he whispers.

This final experience of the story is a multisensory one. Story experiencers are going to see, feel and smell the earth as they plant their acorns; they will be moving and stimulating their proprioceptive and vestibular systems, and perhaps there will even be gentle sound experiences to be had. Gardening is rich in sensory stimuli. It can help to wet the earth you are using with a little warm water – this will give it the feel of warm earth on a summer's day whilst also helping to increase the scent released by the soil as it is manipulated.

You may want to provide small gardening tools, such as a small trowel as even though they are not mentioned in the story itself they may trigger a muscle memory of the action of gardening.

Some people may need physical support to get started – you may want to rest their hands on the earth or move the earth around a little for them as a small demonstration of what can be achieved. It is very important that you remember, and that you ensure anyone else who is helping with the story facilitation knows, that this is about the experience not the goal. What you want is for the person experiencing the story to have the sensory experiences relating to the planting of an acorn in earth. You want for them to touch earth, to smell the soil, to see the change in colours as the earth is disturbed. The aim is not to simply get the acorn planted. This can seem like such an obvious thing to say but often times kind hearted people seeking to 'help' someone view the activity as planting the acorn. They want the person they are supporting to be successful in this activity and so they aid them to plant the acorn as swiftly as possible, rushing them through the experiences they stand most chance of benefiting from.

As this is the last sentence of the story you can let it run for as long as you feel is beneficial. A person experiencing the story may sit with their hands laid passively on top of the tray of soil for five minutes, ten minutes, half an hour before appearing to do anything. Who are we to say what their experience is? Perhaps the touch of the soil connects them with another time when they felt a similar thing, and although they can no longer remember as we understand the word whilst they touch the soil those two experiences of touching connect up in some way for them and so they stay touching to stay connected to that other time. Why would we want to race past that just to get an acorn planted? Other people may take longer to process and understand what is going on; to be gently shown how to push one's hands into the soil, to see it crumble, to lift it and explore it, can be to have a mini sensory adventure. Sometimes after a period of joint exploration like this a person will begin to talk about something that in their mind relates to the experience. It is good to let them talk – wait a while and make sure you understand what is being said, do not assume right away even if what they are saying sounds obvious. If you let them talk you may notice a detail that gives you an extra clue about what it relates to for them.

Sometimes a person will remember how to complete a task through a small sensory warm up, for example if you gently guide their hand to dig with the trowel the motion of digging may connect them with a muscle memory of how to do that task, even though when they looked at the items before them they did not feel as if they were able to do it. Doing is often easier to understand than being shown or instructed. The skill in the facilitation here is to back off as the story experiencer's abilities begin to be revealed. Once again if other people are supporting you in sharing the story it is important you make them aware of the subtleties of facilitating the experience. They may see you digging for someone and think that this is what they should do, when actually what you are doing is more nuanced than that.

After the story is finished you can leave the resources out to be explored. Those story experiencers who have understood the purpose behind the gardener's trip to his garden may be able to talk about how they have or would respond to the birth of a new family member.

Activities to support further engagement with the story

Sensory stories are a great way of introducing a group activity in a care setting, or indeed at home. People delivering, for example, a weekly group activity can feel under pressure to present a different activity each week when actually a good activity repeated is often what people need and respond to best. Using a sensory story to bookend an activity session is a great way of providing consistency of experience and variety, giving the best of both worlds.

To bookend a session with a sensory story simply share the story at the start of the session; it is your cue for the session that is about to take place. Sharing a story together is a great way to generate a sense of connection with the group ahead of joining an activity together. It will gently focus people's attention and if used in this way each week, or each day, it will come to signify to those experiencing it that an active session is about to begin. Once the story is shared – you can move into the activity you have planned, and then as the activity ends come back together to share the story once more. The experiences people have been involved in during the activity may well mean that you see a greater involvement with, or more responses to the story on the second sharing of it.

The following are activities you might wish to use to further support engagement with this story – they are just a few ideas to get you started and you will doubtlessly be able to come up with more.

Planting plants for family members.

Individuals could plant seeds or small plants as gifts to be given to family members. You can do this in a practical or representative way. The practical way to offer this activity is to provide plant pots, soil, seeds or saplings and let people put gifts together for family members. To share this activity in a representative way you provide a person with a large tray of soil and a variety of seeds or nuts to plant. Sitting with them you could gently talk through their family tree, planting a seed or nut for each person as you go. Someone able to access your spoken communication can join you in remembering various family members and patching in anecdotes as you work together to steadily plant the seeds. Someone unable to join you in conversation can join you in the process of planting; they may understand enough of what you say to know the activity is about their family and will welcome the opportunity to be doing something to help. Even if they are not quite sure what the broader picture is of, the simplicity of digging earth and planting seeds should be reassuring. A person unable to access any of the meaning of the conversation can still feel the soil and touch the seeds and at this very sensory level have an interaction with a part of the life cycle of a plant and with life itself. You might choose to display examples of the plants you are planting at different stages of life alongside the activity for people to explore. Having a variety of flowers and branches, small saplings and older plants will add to the sensory atmosphere of the activity and may provide people with prompts to trigger their own minds to reach for pieces of knowledge or scraps of memories.

Decorating plant pots

A very obvious next step to follow on from planting items for family members is to make or decorate plant pots for them to be gifted in. This can be something done over several weeks – perhaps the first week you provide paint for people to paint their plant pot. Although painting a pot can be done quickly it is nice to provide plenty of time for this; a person painting swiftly can paint several pots, someone painting more slowly will be able to complete the activity without feeling like they have been left behind. You can add to the sensory nature of the paint by providing paint of different textures, mixing a little sand with paint will make a gritty texture, or mixing paint to be thick or running. Another way to add sensory interest to the activity of painting is to fragrance the paint. Some paints have strong odours already – it maybe that you can find a variety of paints that have different odours and it is likely that these paint smells will trigger memories of things painted before so you can choose to use them. You will need to use paints like this in a well-ventilated room or outside. Alternatively, find a paint that does not smell too much and add a few drops of essential oils to the mix, you could choose to add scents that match the ones in the story. Try not to use too many otherwise you may find yourself in a room that is a fog of indecipherable smells.

Other steps in decorating pots could include adding a layer of varnish to a design, sticking on small pebbles, shells, buttons or beads, adding a name plate, dipping the rim of the pot in glue and then in glitter or sand to encrust the top of the pot and so on. As an alternative to painting, pots can be decorated with paper wraps which could themselves be drawn upon and decorated whilst flat before being secured around the pot. Wrapping paper to wrap the pots in as gifts could be made by potato printing plain paper or using marbling inks to create a beautiful pattern.

Explore the growth of the child and the tree

In the story the gardener is planting an acorn because his grandchild has just been born. As the child grows so will the acorn, just like the acorn planted on the day of the gardener's birth has grown. You can provide a set of sensory resources to be explored as you chat about this growth.

The acorn and a baby
Possible resources: a single acorn displayed on a empty plate of a contrasting colour. A baby doll. Items associated with very small babies (e.g. nappies, baby wipes, muslin cloths, dummies, rattles). Try to choose resources that would relate to babies that your story experiencer has cared for, this may mean hunting around for older items.

The sapling and the child
Possible resources: a small tree sapling. Small children's clothes, children's toys, building bricks, pull along trucks, train sets and so on. Again if possible hunt for resources that your story experiencer would have played with as a child.

The tree and the adult
Possible resources: a picture of a tree with some tree branches from a similar sized tree displayed alongside. Items associated with adulthood (e.g. car keys, credit cards, handbags, briefcases).

The old tree and the elderly person
Possible resources: a picture of an old tree with some branches from a similar tree displayed alongside. Items associated with later age (e.g. glasses, hearing aids, shawls, pension book, walking stick).

You can share these resources together as a steady conversation of words and experience or you can display them in sequence on a series of small tables or clipped to a washing line along a wall to be explored independently. If sharing them together, remember that the experiences convey meaning in their own right – there does not always need to be words. Allow time for things to be quietly explored.

Discovering seeds or nuts

The gardener took an acorn to plant in his garden, but where did that acorn come from? Did he hunt for it when he was out walking, did he find it in a friend's garden, did he collect it during the previous autumn when it fell from his own oak tree? However it happened the gardener looked for and found the acorn.

Looking for and finding is a task we complete many times a day, often doing it so quickly and so successfully that we hardly recognise it has been done at all. But think of a time when you have looked for something and not found it. How did you feel? Thwarted? Frustrated? Perplexed? Depending on what is lost it can range from very upsetting to simply frustrating to not be able to find an item. Imagine if that did not just happen to you once in a while but repeatedly. It would become not only upsetting and frustrating, but degrading, eroding your self-esteem and your sense of your own abilities. Through your continued failure to find simple things you would quietly lose faith in yourself, your notion of yourself as being a capable person would change, you would consider yourself to be a useless person. When self-esteem drops, it does so exponentially so that at first we feel a little bit bad about ourselves, but then when we meet the next challenge already as someone feeling a bit bad about ourselves and fail again we feel very bad about ourselves, and so meet the next challenge feeling this way and quickly feel astronomically bad about ourselves. This often happens very quietly as someone who thinks ill of themselves is unlikely to assert themselves; the notions of 'I am useless leave me alone' or 'I am useless I am not going to try' are very easily acquired.

If you are sharing this story with someone who appears to be a passive recipient they could well hold these sad ideas about their personal worth inside of themselves. Something so simple it almost seems not to be a task at all, like looking for and finding an acorn, can be a way to counter that creeping sense of personal failure inside of them.

The task is simple, and the resources likewise, you are going to be looking for and finding acorns. My advice would be to begin with a version of this that you are confident will be too easy for the person you are offering it to and then step up gradually but stop before failure.

Gradations of the task could include:

- an acorn on a plate of contrasting colour, with a request to be passed the acorn

- an acorn on a plate that is patterned or brown in colour, with a request to be passed the acorn

- an acorn on a plate or in a deep sided tray that has shredded paper sprinkled lightly over the top such that the acorn can still be clearly seen through it (using a contrasting colour of paper is helpful here)

- an acorn in a box or a deep sided tray with shredded paper heaped on top of it. The colour of the shredded paper could be varied to increase the challenge

- an acorn in a box or pot with leaves laid over the top of it

- an acorn in a box or pot sprinked with earth, or buried in earth.

You can also use the different resources in this exploration to vary the sensory experiences you are offering to people – garden centres have a variety of wood mulches or even gravel chips that could be used to hide acorns.

In all of the explorations you are going to be asking people to find an acorn for you and then responding with the gratitude the gardener would have shown one of his friends if they had found the perfect acorn for him to use to record the birth of his grandchild.

Tray gardens

Of course one of the best things you could do in response to this story is step outside into your own garden and do a spot of gardening. However not everyone has a garden, or nice weather for gardening in, and not everyone can step outside as they might wish to, and so tray gardens can be offered as an alternative.

Deep-sided trays can be used to create small gardens and the opportunities to be creative with this activity are endless; for example, you could create a small moss garden, collecting moss from walls and trees and laying it onto damp earth to grow. Kept moist it will stay alive. You could grow quick-growing seeds such as cress on a thin layer of damp earth. Or you could go down the zen garden route and fill your tray with sand or tiny gravel particles and relax by laying pebbles down in patterns or raking through it with a small rake.

Exploring perfumes

As the gardener steps into his garden he pauses to appreciate the smell of the different flowers. Exploring scents is a lovely way to hold a sensory conversation, but take it slowly as they can be very powerful connectors and very emotional to memory. Avoid overwhelming people by placing resources a little way apart so that people travel through clear air between smells, or by pacing your delivery of the smells such that there are times when people are smelling a scent with pauses between when the air is clear – perhaps have a window open to ensure you are not just filling the room up with layer upon layer of odour.

The nicest way to explore floral smells would be with fresh cut flowers. These would also be a visual delight. A room set with wide-based vases (such that they are hard to knock over) each displaying a single fresh flower would be a delight to explore. Other options would be potpourri, essential oils, perfumes, or toiletries.

Bark rubbings

The gardener rests his hand against the bark of the old tree feeling its texture. Using wax crayons to take rubbings of different textured surfaces is a way to explore texture through touch and sight. Taking a rubbing is simple, you just lay a piece of paper over the surface you wish to rub and, using the crayon on its side so that a long flat edge rests on the paper, you rub it against the paper-covered object. The texture of the object will be revealed in the pattern emerging on the paper.

To support people in taking rubbings ensure the object being rubbed is well secured. Going outside and holding paper against trees is one way to ensure a bark rubbing in which the bark does not slip away from you. If you are taking rubbings indoors using something like a silicone baking sheet to create a nonslip surface on a table onto which to place the bark can be a handy way to assist someone. Another alternative is to use simple D clips (these can be purchased inexpensively from high street shops) to secure the bark to the table.

Leaf mobiles

The gardener stands below the leaf canopy of the tree grown from the acorn planted on the day of his birth. The pattern of leaves above our heads is one of nature's great beauties and exploring the leaves themselves is a way to be drawn in to the extraordinary intricacies of these everyday objects.

Creating a leaf mobile is a good vehicle for exploring leaves. It maybe you are supporting someone who could create their own leaf mobile, but more likely you will be supporting someone for whom making a mobile would be too fiddly, therefore it will be your job to thread leaves onto cotton and tie them off and then attach these threads perhaps to a wire coat hanger so that they form a simple mobile. The person you are supporting will be tasked with choosing the best leaves from a selection you present. As with all the tasks do not get muddled as to what the point of this task is, and ensure that anyone else supporting you in delivering the activity is clear too. The point is the sensory exploration and engagement with the natural materials. The point is not to create a mobile. If a mobile gets created, super; if it does not, then that does not matter a jot.

A natural sort

I imagine the gardener's garden to be very well looked after, perhaps it looks wild to the untrained eye but each plant is carefully tended or perhaps it is one of those incredibly neat gardens where plants are sorted by height and colour to fit perfectly into their surroundings.

Sorting things out, creating order out of chaos, however small the scale, can have therapeutic benefits. Offering a story experiencer a selection of natural resources to spend time contemplating and sorting is a simple but effective task. Think about when you last sat on a beach with a little time to spare. Did you sift through the sand around you, selecting pebbles or shells that took your fancy and laying these out in your lap or on your towel? Perhaps you even took them home because they seemed precious to you and now serve to remind you of that time sat on the beach.

The key to making this task appealing is in the presentation of the resources. Think of the nature of the surface you will spread the resources out upon and how this will contribute to their appeal and appearance. Options you might consider which offer visual and tactile appeal are: wooden surfaces, grass – fake or real – a swathe of velvet fabric, a plain table cloth, a slate placemat and so on. You could even present some resources beautifully on a tray covered in water – this works especially well for stones or shells. Another alternative to this is to rub a little olive oil onto pebbles or shells, or even the surface of leaves, before laying them out for exploration – the oil will add a little gloss to the objects, making them visually more appealing. Think also about how you will light the work area – a table in a window, or well lit with a lamp will make objects look more appealing. By following links from www.TheSensoryProjects.co.uk to Facebook you can access public photo albums containing all sorts of sensory inspiration, among them one with instructions for making an improvised light box which can also be employed to make objects for exploration look visually appealing.

You can inspire people to begin to sort resources by showing them the work of artists who employ material sorting in their works; for example, Andy Goldsworthy's amazing leaf artworks or James Eddy's charcoal sculptures. You may need to sit with a person and slowly sift the resources with them. Try not to make this sifting target based; do not sit with them and begin to organise leaves into a colour fading line or arrange stones in a geometric pattern as doing this imposes your ideas on their exploration. You might sit with them and manipulate the resources, maybe make a little space and begin to lay a few items down in this space, perhaps commenting on shape or colour, or you could hand them a leaf or a pebble to look at. Your investigations act as a warm up for their own movements and explorations.

Summary: sensory stories

Sensory stories are a simple and rewarding way of sharing a sensory conversation. Packaging experiences into a story makes the overall experience more engaging than the sum of its parts whilst also providing story experiencers with access to the richness of narrative.

Section 6

Sensory support

Orientation

Having an understanding of the sensory world can help you to re-evaluate everyday situations and introduce forms of sensory support for the person for whom you care. This section looks at how you can offer sensory support for life skills, for joining in with an activity, for orientating a person and also for addressing sensory confusion. We also look at how we can use this knowledge to create a flight path for someone experiencing the sort of distress that may lead to violent outbursts.

Practical: sensory support for life skills

At the start of this book I used an analogy of a person sending messages through a forest to someone on the other side to represent what the experience of living with a brain which has dementia might be like. In one of these analogies I described lots of different messengers setting out through that forest of a mind but only some getting through.

As a person attempts to navigate their own life, completing tasks we take for granted like going to the kitchen to make a drink of water or getting dressed involves drawing on lots of different sets of knowledge. A person making a drink may be seated and engaged in a different activity when they think about getting a drink; it may be that they think to get a drink because they feel the sensation of thirst and know that this represents a need in their body for water, it maybe that they think about getting a drink because they are aware that it is healthy to be hydrated and have made a commitment to themselves to drink more water. Both of these motivators for getting a drink are based on knowledge held within the mind, the first on the knowledge that thirst indicates a lack of hydration and the second on the knowledge that hydration is important. Once they have decided to get a drink they get up and navigate their way to the kitchen; to do this they use an internal map they have of their house and their senses of sight and touch to find the route. In the kitchen they locate a cup from within the cupboard, they know to find the cup there because they have a memory of where the cups are kept, and they turn on the tap holding the cup beneath it to fill it.

I have skipped over many of the details involved in getting a drink but from my brief overview of the process you can see that it is much more than simply getting a drink. A person who gets up to get a drink relies on a variety of current sensory experiences and chunks of remembered knowledge to complete the task. The person you are supporting may be missing some of these things, and to complete that simple task of getting a drink without them is a little bit like asking a clockwork clock to complete the simple task of turning its second hand once around the face but without one tiny cog. It is only one cog, so what does it matter? It matters enormously!

We can use sensory experiences to support this person in maintaining their own independence. This is not something we are looking to do just because we cannot be bothered to fetch the glass of water for them, far from it. This is something we are looking to do because we recognise how valuable being able to fetch that glass of water for themselves is, not only for that person's physical wellbeing but for their mental wellbeing as well. Jakob and Collier (2014) tell us that stimulation and activity appropriate to the individual will help to keep them active and included. In enabling them to fetch the glass of water for themselves we enable them to play an active and positive role in their own lives which is a fantastically valuable thing to do. We can help them to do that by using our knowledge of what makes for strong sensory experiences to give them extra messages to support their carrying out of the task.

Imagine that forest again – in a mind that is fully functional the message to get a glass of water is sent and passes swiftly through a network of forest paths, taking in the knowledge points, accessing the sensory stimuli and successfully completing the task. In a mind that has been changed by dementia that messenger sets off, but as she walks confidently along the path she has walked many times before suddenly it appears different, she is disorientated, she gets stuck and gets no further. Offering supportive sensory experiences does not fix those blocks but does provide additional messages to support that original messenger when she encounters blocks along her route. In essence we will be filling that forest with extra messengers who can, when the original messenger gets lost, step out from the bushes and guide her to the next part of her route so that she can continue on again until the next time she gets lost when hopefully someone else will step forward and take him to the next step.

In your physical support of the person you will be doing the same – maybe they need help to get up from the chair; you will give them that help but then withdraw your support; you will not support them all the way to the tap. Maybe they will successfully get the cup from the cupboard and hold it under the tap, but not turn the tap on; you will turn the tap on or take their hand to the head of the tap and begin the turn with them, and then withdraw your support. What you do not want to do is see their intent to get a drink, see them struggling, and then just do it for them. Remember the forest, if a part of the path is missing and you can get them through that then they can continue to tread the rest of the path and maintain it. If you take over the whole task then the remainder of that path in their mind is likely to become overgrown and unnavigable.

How do we use strong sensory experiences to help a person complete a task which they cannot fully do independently? First we must think about that task through each of our senses, attempting to disregard the cognitive information we rely upon to complete the task. So, for example, what does getting a drink look like?

Well initially getting a drink does not look like anything at all! So this is an obvious place we can improve things. What if when suggesting to someone that they get a drink we placed an empty glass down in front of them, or even handed them a photo of a full glass of water. In this way as the task begins there is a visual cue for what is to be done.

Moving forward in the task, getting a drink looks like the route from wherever the person was at the start of this endeavour to wherever the water is located that will become their drink. Most likely this is a route through a few rooms, perhaps out of the living room along a corridor and into the kitchen. What does this route look like? Are there clear visual markers to help a person navigate? These could include door frames painted in a bold contrasting colour, or dado rails to act as connecting lines between doors. Are there visual markers that might work against a person trying to move from where they are to where they can get a drink? These could include patterned carpets which people with dementia can find alarming to walk across or bright visual distractions in the environment around.

At the final stage of the task getting a drink looks like the cupboard with the cup in and the tap. Looking at a cupboard does not really tell you much about cups and taps. A simple way to support this step would be to have a cup out in the kitchen already near to the tap. Using a glass or clear plastic beaker adds extra support as the person pouring the water can see when it is nearing the top from the sides as well as from on top.

Once you have assessed the visual strengths and weaknesses of each stage of the process involved in getting a drink you can go about sorting them out. Draw on the information on visual stimulus in Section 4 to support you in choosing clear visual messages to send.

Then repeat this process for each of the other senses, paying particular attention to those you feel the person you are looking to support is particularly responsive. A few sensory tweaks may make the difference between someone being dependent on you and someone being able to function independently. I have begun with our visual sense because we are a sight-dominated society but you may well be supporting someone whose sight is impaired in some way; for this person it will be especially important to attend to the information provided by the other sensory systems.

Below is a brief overview of some of the things you might be taking into account as you consider this example. Of course this is just an example in a book; you might be looking to support someone in doing something completely different, perhaps it is getting into the car and putting their seat belt on, or taking their clothes out of a cupboard and putting them on. There are so many options I could not possibly detail them all here. What I hope to do is set your brain thinking in a sensory way and then you will be able to do the sensory detective work necessary to put in sensory support for a person and remove any sensory input likely to thwart their independence.

Olfactory experiences

Do the different rooms in a location have different smells? Can scent be used to orientate someone to where they are. Often kitchens have a distinct odour and so do bathrooms (hopefully a pleasant one as a result of well-chosen cleaning products). Other rooms can come to have smells associated with them; rooms with lots of soft furnishings may hold the smell of the fabric conditioner used upon them, scented candles or plug in air fresheners also add fragrance to a room.

Gustatory experiences

If you use a glass to represent going to get a drink at the start of the process, having a single sip of water in it can be an extra prompt – the person tasting the water can then be asked to get more. The reverse of this is that if someone is currently engaged in a different gustatory experience this may fill the attention of this sense such that it does not consider desiring the taste of water.

Tactile experiences

Having a cup to hold as you travel to get water can be a reminder of what it is that you are up to every step of the way. A person beginning a journey from one location to another in order to get water may get distracted by something else along the way and forget what it was they were doing; if they are touching something that reminds them of their task they will be quicker to orientate than if they find themselves in a location with no clues as to their previous purpose.

Auditory experiences

Do the different rooms have different sounds? Will a person moving from one room to another experience sounds that distract or distress them along the way? Will you be providing auditory prompts as they seek to complete their task? Is the general soundscape of the environment calming in which concentration and memory are going to be fostered or a more distressing one where concentration and memory will be hampered?

A great example of settings using sensory support for independence is the growing number giving their residents the chance to decorate their zimmer frames in a multisensory way.[1] These settings have found that enabling residents to decorate their zimmer frames with bright colours, with textures, and even with things that make a noise as they move, is a way of supporting them in remembering to use their frames. The increased use of the frames has contributed to reduced rates of injury with one setting reporting a 60 per cent drop in the number of falls. The heightened sensory nature of the frames draws attention to them and helps residents to distinguish their own zimmer frame from someone else's, thus avoiding the problems that may occur from walking off with someone else's frame. A nice addition to this is that often times people's names are a part of the decoration, meaning that people encountering them who may not otherwise know their names are able to use them which in turn contributes to a friendlier setting.

---

1   https://www.carehome.co.uk/news/article.cfm/id/1582010/Pimped-up-Zimmer-frames

---

Sensory support for involvement in an activity

If you are looking to share an activity with an individual with dementia or with a group of individuals with dementia, doing a sensory audit of how you have set up the activity space and how you are going to guide people to it can be very helpful in generating maximum engagement with the task.

This is essentially the same process as described in the example above about getting a glass of water. You are going to consider how each aspect of what you will be doing is presented through each of the sensory systems. I would suggest focusing on three things:

1. the layout of the environment in which the activity will take place

2. the sensory nature of the activity itself

3. the sensory aspects of the journey to the activity, including being informed about the activity taking place.

You can use the information about sensory experiences in Section 4 to inform your audit of each of these things.

For the environment think about how you will present a clear sensory focus on the activity you are offering. Here is an example of visual support for an activity.

The activity is a making task. The choice of location is a relatively sparse room. The activity is laid out on a large table which has been spread with a plain red table cloth. The resources of white paper plates, white glue sticks and sparkly paper stand out well in contrast to the table cloth. The chairs in the room have all been orientated to point towards the table. Other items that offered visual stimulus have been removed from the room or draped over with sheets (e.g. a bright display board).

The layout described above sends a clear visual message as to what is going to be happening. Whereas a room with several tables, each supporting something different – one the resources for the activity, another some paper work, another some bits and bobs belonging to someone in the room, and the chairs still in their usual locations waiting to be drawn up to the table with the resources on – sends a confused visual message.

As with Sensory Support for Independence you will think through each of the sensory systems as you plan the set up of the activity. Consider having a sensory focus for each of the sensory systems within the activity, and then removing competing stimuli from the room where possible.

In considering the sensory journey to the activity you will be considering the same things as we explored in the earlier example of a person getting a glass of water. So we are left with the sensory presentation of the activity itself. Again we are looking at using the same skill of evaluating the sensory experiences present and working out how to clarify these so that they send easy to interpret supporting messages for what is expected of a person within the activity, but you are doing this in greater detail.

The precise sensory support you offer within an activity will be tailored to the activity and the people you are sharing it with. Here are a few examples:

Dennis is partially sighted; he is taking part in an activity that involves threading buttons onto string. The staff supporting Dennis have looked at ways of giving him tactile support for this activity. They gave Dennis a shoe lace to thread the buttons onto, the top of the lace is wrapped in a plastic sheath to prevent it from fraying, and this gives Dennis's fingers something hard and pointy to hold onto which is easier for him than the wool other participants are using. The buttons Dennis is using for his threading are brightly coloured, flat, shiny and hard, they have been laid out on Dennis' table on neutral-coloured rough hessian matting which presents both a visual and tactile contrast to the buttons, making it easy for Dennis to locate them and pick them up.

Anjali often appears not to hear people – the staff in her setting are unsure as to whether this is caused by her dementia or by a degeneration in her hearing. Every Thursday afternoon a sing-song is organised in the living room. Anjali usually attends but appears passive. The team member leading the session decided to try something a little bit creative and purchased half a dozen sound tubes from a local shop for just over five pounds. They led a call and response session using these tubes to support interaction. They delivered the call into the end of the tube and held the other end to a resident's ear, and then moved the end they had called into to be in front of the resident's mouth like a microphone ready for their response. Having the tube held near their ear meant that for these residents the call was presented straight to their ear, making it stand out more boldly against the background noise of the setting. Some residents were able to make the response back into the tube and Anjali appeared more engaged than normal.

Sensory support flight path

By pulling together the insights you have gained from the support strategies above with the information in the vocabulary section of Section 4 you probably already have a good idea of how to create a flight path. Refer back to the example of the cat I gave in Section 2. You can create a flight path for someone if you regularly support them in a particular environment. A flight path needs to end in a safe space – some of the small environment spaces discussed in Section 7 may be suitable; other safe spaces could be a person's bed, or a particular chair where they know they will be not be intruded upon.

In order to be effective the flight path needs to be clearly defined, regularly used (even when not in fight or flight) and must lead to somewhere where the person you are supporting feels safe. If they already have a place they escape to do not try and change it. If that place is inappropriate in some way then try and solve that problem rather than attempt to create a whole new space for them. If they do not currently have a safe space try to create one. It will need to look familiar; they will probably respond well to a small dimly lit space, and having appealing comforting items in the space can also be beneficial.

The route to that space needs to be clear to the senses. This sounds simple, but nevertheless it is important to think carefully about the path to the safe place. If there is a light that flashes along that route, or if there are loud sudden sounds that occur as someone is travelling along that route – perhaps shouted instructions, perhaps sound from things collided with – or even just if there is an object blocking the path, like a chair pulled out or a bag on the floor, all of these things can – in a situation of stress – act a little like the straw that broke the camel's back – they will be the final piece of aggravation that turns flight into fight.

If you are supporting someone who is regularly expressing themselves through violence think about where they are when that happens. Does it tend to be around particular activities, or is it at particular times of the day or in particular places? You may be recognising that it is happening during activities that in themselves provide a lot of sensory stimulation – perhaps this is too much for the person – in this case you will be thinking less about flight paths and more about how you can reduce the stimulation of the activities. Sometimes just slowing a routine down can help so that brushing one's teeth does not come immediately after having one's hair dried and so on. Or you may be able to think of ways to mitigate the sensory distress (e.g. by playing music to cover the noise of an electronic toothbrush and the running water).

If violence is an occurrence that happens not necessarily in response to a particular stimulus or situation but just as part of the very understandable build up of frustration that people experiencing dementia feel, then consider where that person typically is and where they could flee to. If they spend their days in the living room can they flee to a bedroom, or to a quiet corner of the garden? It needs to be somewhere they will be safe on their own. Try to teach them this flight path – when you notice their agitation growing walk them along the path to the safe place and leave them there to calm down. Do this as a supporter not a disciplinarian. You are not walking a child to a naughty step, you are guiding an adult to a place of sanctuary. The safe space is a gift to them not a punishment. Your repeated support of them in accessing the place will make them more likely to take the flight path you have laid out when they encounter a distressing situation.

All behaviour is communication. People are not violent without reason. A person turning to violence to express themselves is likely to be under a great deal of stress and to have run out of alternative expression strategies. Even if to you it may seem as if nothing has provoked the violence, it is worth considering again how the situation may appear to the person you are supporting.

The sensory world is just one lens to look through as you do your detective work. Was there a sensory stimulus or an overload of stimulus that prompted the violence? Do not rely on your own senses to inform you of this – it is all too easy to assume that our own sensory perceptions are an authority on everyone else's. We can judge whether a room is too hot or too cold; we know whether a light is too bright or too dim *for us*, and for us alone. We do not know what someone else's senses are telling them. Dementia damages nerve cells in the brain preventing them from communicating with each other and eventually destoying them. Some forms of dementia can cause blockages in cells in the brain. No part of the brain is protected from dementia so this damage can be done to the parts of the brain that process sensory information. The person you are supporting may receive certain sensory messages much louder than you or much weaker, their abilities to perceive and understand sensory information may fluctuate and they could be experiencing sensory hallucinations. Look for clues in how they respond to help you to evaluate whether there may be a sensory influence at play; for example, if they screw their eyes up or clap their hands to their ears this would indicate them trying to block out stimulus. To be clear: I am not saying that all outbursts of violence have a sensory cause, an outburst could just as easily be caused by a fear about an upcoming event (e.g. being asked to get into a car when you do not understand where the car is going). Nevertheless the senses are worth considering as you seek to understand their behaviour. Try not to simply write off a violent episode as for no reason at all. Doing this dismisses your own right to safety as well as their distress. You are both precious and you should both be able to feel safe.

Independent sensory activities

An independent sensory activity is something that a person with dementia can access at a sensory level and be engaged in without support. Fiddle blankets and twiddle muffs are good examples of this sort of activity but we can create an independent sensory activity out of almost anything if we use our knowledge of what makes things interesting to the senses (see sensory vocabulary in Section 4 for ideas).

Blankets, cushions and muffs

Sensory blankets, cushions or muffs all use fabric or knit to create a familiar object onto which are stitched items of sensory interest. Often times groups seeking to do good in their community will produce these. In my community the team of a local supermarket knit twiddle muffs during their breaks and the local Women's Institute group makes fiddle blankets to donate to our local hospice and hospital. The people who create these items are keen to make them as interesting and engaging as possible but may lack the sensory knowledge to make the most out of their efforts. If you are able to give them some guidance you will get an even better resource. So, for example, people may not look to include hard, sharp objects on their creations, even though these are likely to provide tactile interest. You can explain that the rough side of Velcro® or the pointy part of a press stud might improve their creations. Here are a few more examples of things that are good to include on a fabric-based sensory activity (I would not necessarily put all of these on one item, that could overwhelm, rather I would look to make a few items that each offer different opportunities for engagement):

- **Photo keyrings.** You can buy keyring fobs that allow you to slide a photo of a family member or favourite item inside – these can be interesting for people to browse.

- **Fluorescent colours against dark plain backdrops.** These will provide points of bold visual interest. You could use a fluorescent thread to pick out a shape that is meaningful to the individual for whom the resource is for (e.g. the shape of a favourite flower or the outline of a pet).

- **Rough, hard, sharp, cold things!** Including these items is counterintuitive initially, but against fabric they provide an interesting tactile contrast. Belt buckles are hard, cold and have the sharp point of the buckle. Rough Velcro®, or rough fabrics like hessian offer a tactile contrast to softer fabrics like fur and velvet. Stiffened fabrics, for example the webbing used in the top of curtains, also offer contrast. A trip to your local haberdashers will reveal a wealth of options, but remember not to be drawn in to choosing with your vision alone.

- **Elastic** that can be pulled against offers resistance through the joints and in so doing stimulates the proprioceptive system. Pinging things on elastic is always fun too.

- **Bells and scrunches.** Look for ways to add sounds to a resource – bells are an obvious way to do this. For an alternative stitch scrunchy plastic or foil inside a resource so that when it is manipulated the foil or plastic scrunches.

- **Zip mesh wash bags.** These are sold to protect delicates in the wash; they are small nylon mesh bags that fasten with a zip; they can be easily stitched onto a resource and then the pouch can be used to hold items that may need to be refreshed or removed for washing. They are great way to include a scent on a fabric resource. I have made a little pouch of coffee beans and popped them inside the bag and have also had lots of fun with different herbal tea bags. These release a gentle aroma, strong enough to be accessed by someone close by, and are wonderfully easy to replenish.

Small tasks, such as:

- **Zips** to do up and unzip. Support these by attaching loops to the zip head to make them easier to pull or better yet a loop with a bead or button threaded onto it to make it easier to grip.

- **Buttons** with matching button holes.

- **Toggles** with loops.

All of these small tasks would once have been part of a much bigger, more elaborate task that perhaps now cannot be done, but done in isolation they are a way of drip feeding small achievements to a person and in this way are supportive of their self-esteem. Think about the sensory nature of each – choose buttons that stand out against the fabric they are stitched too either in colour or texture, ensure that button holes or loops are big enough to be spotted and manipulated with ease. Consider using a contrasting stitch colour to highlight the button hole.

- **Chair tidy.** An individual with dementia may spend a lot of time seated; this can be because of co-occurring physical disabilities or frailties or it can be as a result of the situation in which they find themselves. If you are supporting a more active person with dementia there may be times when you wish for them to be seated for their own safety; for example, perhaps you feel more confident about their wellbeing if they are sat in a safe place whilst you go and take a shower than if they are roaming around the house. In both of these scenarios having chair-based sensory activities can be an asset to the care you are providing. Chair tidies are sold to house the various remote controls, pens, paper, newspapers and puzzle books that often surround our chairs at home. They hang over the arm of a chair such that their pockets rest against the outer side of the chair.

Think about the things typically in these pockets: puzzle books, of interest if your brain is able to work out puzzles; newspapers, of interest if you are able to read and follow the news; remote controls, useful if you can see well enough to work out which button is which and then a route to entertainment only if you are able to process the audio and visual information outputted at speed by the television. A lot of people without dementia struggle to process information at the speed television demands, and I would argue that it is rarely an interesting experience for someone with dementia.

We are going to look to replace these items with things that will hold sensory interest.

The sensory equivalent to a puzzle book might be a large match-box (without matches); this offers a rough edge, a distinctive smell, when one end is depressed the other opens – which is a little puzzle in itself, and then inside the matchbox what is there to discover? Perhaps a few sweets, perhaps an interesting object or a crunched up sheet of coloured cellophane.

The sensory equivalent to a television control could be a sensory toy that lights up and produces sound when buttons on it are pressed – this could be a vibrant loud bright item or something gentler and more soothing. There are any number of such things on the market, look for ones with buttons that are clear and easy to press.

The sensory equivalent to a newspaper could be an item that reports on news personal to that person; for example, a photo of a recent visitor, an object from a recent trip, or even something simple like the paper cup that was drunk from on a visit to a café. These all report news in a sensory way.

If you make your own chair tidy you might choose to have the pockets hang on the inside of the chair arm so that they are more easily noticed. If you are using a shop-bought chair tidy with pockets that hang down the outside of the chair's arm you might opt to clip something bright to the top to draw attention over the arm of the chair, or you could even attach some things to coloured ribbons and drape these ribbons into the inside of the chair to be noticed, explored and possibly pulled upon revealing the object below.

An alternative to a chair tidy can be a pocketed apron – you can buy tabards with a single big pocket on the front which can work. Even better are aprons with multiple pockets. You could wear such an item laden with sensory wonders to hold a sensory conversation with someone or you could make a personalised one for an individual which would enable to wearer to have easy access to a range of sensory wonders as and when they liked. Another portable option is a fisherman's vest, or any garment with a lot of pockets – these can be loaded with items of sensory interest for the wearer to discover.

Wash rolls – travel washbags that unroll to hang on the back of a bathroom door or inside a shower as a small portable bathroom cabinet – are easily available and great for storing a small sensory conversation inside. These are wonderful for sensory work as they are often splendidly decorated – you can find a bright eye catching one in a style to suit the person you are supporting, or you might opt for a more sophisticated darker coloured one as a stylish way of carrying sensory items around to support someone. Use your knowledge of the person you are creating this sensory conversation for to inform your choice of what to put into the roll. Bathroom products can be a good source of stimuli: a flavoured lip balm to stimulate taste, a hand rub or scrub for tactile, proprioceptive and olfactory stimulation, wash mitts, exfoliation gloves or loofahs for rough tactile stimulation. Of course you do not have to use bathroom resources, the sturdy and generally water proof nature of these bags makes them suitable for housing all sorts of resources. The bag's hook or loop makes them great for moving around and displaying; for example, a wheelchair user can have their own personalised set of sensory resources easily hung on the back of their chair. The bag can be hung easily from the back of another chair drawn up in front of someone for them to explore.

Mini string – sequence strings were discussed at the end of Section 4. A mini string can be easily created from a coat hanger by clipping things along the horizontal bar of the hanger. Other options include draping a small piece of netting over someone's knees and clipping items to this, using safety pins to secure a thread across a scatter cushion, or hanging a thread and creating a vertical string. I would advise not making vertical strings too strong; it is highly unlikely that anyone would get their neck caught up in one but if they did you would want the string to pull free of its tether point long before it became a danger to anyone.

A fidget board or box – Fidget boxes or boards can be thought of as the rigid alternative to fabric fidget items; they are wooden sensory blankets. When you were thinking about creating a fabric resource I suggested a visit to your local haberdashers and viewing things through sensory eyes. For a fidget board I recommend a trip to your local DIY shop with your senses alert to the possibilities. The aisles of a DIY store are a sensory paradise: different grades of sandpaper, chains and links that clank and cling, locks and catches that can be done and undone, drip feeding self-esteem as they go. Bright paints, matt paints, chalk, fairy lights, door bells, buzzers, coloured tiles with different textures, textured wall paper, reflective tape, the list goes on and on. Normally people visit a DIY store with a plan in mind – there is something at home that needs fixing and they have come to the store to find the items required for the job. Viewed in that way they can seem rather dull places. Visit one with sensory stimulation in mind, walk the aisles thinking 'What makes a noise, what different sounds can I find?' 'What do things feel like, how many textures can I find' and you will quickly realise you are in a sensory wonderland. Buy one of everything (in so far as you can afford it) and secure them to a wooden board or box and you will have a fabulous sensory fiddle resource.

If you do not have the woodworking skills or tools required for creating the sort of board described above much can be achieved with strong cardboard, double-sided sticky tape and cable ties.

Familiar sensory objects – if you know the person whom you are supporting well, then you may have insight into their life and know what sorts of items they are likely to have encountered through their lives. If you do not know them that well you may be able to speak to a family member or loved one who could give you this insight. Finding objects that the person you are supporting relates to tidying up and sorting things can give you the 'in' for an activity. If when they see the item they associate it with having to *do* something then this association can be the catalyst for them getting started in an activity and often getting started is the trickiest thing.

Here are a few examples: desk tidies, cutlery drawer inserts, mug stands, shoe tidies, hooks, jewellery boxes,[2] even chocolate boxes.

Tidying the items intended to be tidied into these objects is often a sensory activity which you can add a little extra sensory sparkle to. For example, someone putting shoes onto a shoe rack could be offered sparkly ballet slippers, pointy high heels, grubby work boots and smelly trainers – quite a sensory assortment. But you do not have to restrict yourself to the items normally sorted into these objects.

---

2   Many companies now do ranges of sensory jewellery. This can be jewellery that is suitable for chewing on as a stress reliever, jewellery that has some naturally fiddly component to toy with, or jewellery that creates sound by jingling or chiming. If you are using a jewellery box to support someone perhaps an investment in sensory jewellery would not go amiss!

For example, the insert of a chocolate box could be used to display different flower heads, or coloured pompoms. By offering a mixture of items, some heavy, some light, some bright, some dull, some sound making, others silent you quickly make a small sensory activity with a lot of different notes of interest within it.

Treasure box

Boxes are wonderful for all their practical properties, i.e. they can look beautiful and they are very very handy for keeping things inside, but also for more subtle valuable properties concerned with the preservation of our mental wellbeing when we find ourselves accessing knowledge and understanding of the world in a very sensory way. For some people as their journey into dementia progresses they may find themselves with very little ability to understand life the way it is and to anticipate a future. Our ability to hope and to feel positive about life is based in our understanding of time and our understanding of change. To feel hope we need to know that there is a future time and we need to know that it is possible for things to be different in that time to how they are now. Trying to break the concept of hope down, even here in this simple way, very quickly becomes complex. Trying to persuade someone to feel hopeful or feel positive when they are losing their orientation in the world and their understanding of it is very very difficult for everyone involved. But boxes are a small part of it! That's why they are so amazing.

Someone who sees a box and looks to open it is someone who is using their knowledge of the world to see a future – a future where the box is opened, they know that the opening of the box can happen and in this they know change is possible. When they look inside the box to see what is there, that is a looking forward into the future. It is on a micro scale, but when you have so little left micro scales are all the more precious.

It is very easy when you are supporting someone who accesses the world and meaning within it in a sensory way to give them the sensory items that engage them as a fait accompli – to just hand them the item so that in their experience it was just there.

Perhaps their engagement and interest in the world was triggered by the item, so prior to the item being there they were not really aware and then you put it down and suddenly it was there and they were interested. To the person in this experience the world just is as it is; they are not linking up the moment before the item was given to them with the item being passed to them, they are not understanding that change is coming ahead of it coming, they are just there and life is either interesting or it is not and there is nothing they can do about it.

If you bring that fascinating item over to the person inside a box or a bag, and try to gain their interest as you open that box or bag, perhaps in time they learn that the item they love is kept in that box or bag and then when they see the box or bag they anticipate change; they reach in their mind into the future, and the future they reach to is a positive one. It is a little rehearsal of hope, an exercising of the thoughts that keep those positive neural pathways through the mind open.

As well as making the 'reveal' a part of any sensory conversation, providing someone beginning on their sensory adventures with boxes to explore keeps alive their natural curiosity in the world and excitement about possibilities yet to come. Hunting for great boxes is a lot of fun. I find friends often keep good boxes they have come across or brightly coloured paper bags and pass them on to me. They enjoy doing this and I enjoy being the recipient of the strange gifts and the people I pass them onto enjoy exploring them. It makes me smile to think of the friend in a suit doing a busy high flying office job and stopping in their march across the office because they have noticed a fancy bag on someone else's desk and want to enquire if they can have it for me.

Once you have got the interesting boxes or bags you know what to do with them! Find something wonderful to put inside, wonderful for its sensory richness and then do a quick assessment of what sensory support is available for opening the box or bag. Is the opening obvious? If the box is beautifully decorated with a pattern that joins up perfectly across the seam upon which it opens then the addition of some bright coloured sticky tape will sort that out. Can you staple on a tag or tie that will make the box or bag easier to open? Natural items are super for putting in these boxes and quick to find, a few leaves from a tree, some fruit from the shop, a fir cone, or a feather.

Summary: sensory support

Thinking about how we communicate in a sensory way can facilitate offering support to an individual with dementia. By offering sensory support we can enable someone with dementia: to carry out basic life skill tasks such as making a cup of tea; engage in an activity; escape from situations where they feel unsafe; and take part in independent sensory activities.

Section 7

Sensory environments

Orientation

The environment within which a sensory exchange takes place is just as critical to that exchange's success as is the choice of stimuli and facilitation of the exchange itself. People with dementia are very sensitive to sensory experience so their environment needs to be carefully managed (Behrman *et al.* 2014). By considering the sensory nature of the environments we occupy, and also by creating bespoke sensory environments to support the needs of individuals with dementia, we can enrich their lives and enhance the connection we are able to make with them.

Standing out

Choosing the right sensory stimuli for a sensory conversation is important but just as important is the environment in which you share that stimuli. It will be as difficult for someone to focus on a small photograph in a brightly decorated room as it would be for you to listen to the words spoken by a friend in amidst a cacophony of other voices. Think about how the environment we are in distracts from the stimuli we are sharing, or contrasts with it – thus making it stand out more boldly. This is as important a consideration as the general atmosphere of the environment itself.

In this section you will find creative ideas for sensory environments of increasing size, beginning with small portable

environments and ending with considerations of wider environments outside of our control.

Small sensory spaces

Small environments can be a great way of fostering engagement.
We feel safer in small spaces, and it is our natural instinct when in
danger to seek out a small hidey hole. Someone in a large space
can be in a state of alert, subconsciously checking for danger all
the while and distracted and agitated because of this. In a small
space that energy that was taken up with checking for danger can
be redirected into your conversation.

A natural small space to create is the corner of a room, or simply
convert a small room in a house. Consider the sensory properties
you are looking for when it comes to providing a small sensory
space, these are likely to be the sensory experiences that support
people to feel calm, and refer to the sensory vocabulary in Section 4
to remind yourself of what these might be.

Considering things like curtains, cushions and lighting can all
have a big effect on the sensory environment in a small room.
Use lightweight curtains to mute the light in the room, rather
than fill the room with harsh bright light. Adding cushions or
other soft furnishings will absorb sound in the room and so soften
the auditory environment as well as the tactile. Using fairy lights
or fibre optic displays (which can be cheaply purchased online)
adds visual interest without overwhelming. Think about what the
person you are supporting will want to do in the room, is it a
place where they will come to in order to relax and calm down,
i.e. a place where you are essentially looking for them to be still
and unwind rather than to be active and engaged? Or is it a place
where they will come in order to gain focus and attune themselves
to an activity? Your purpose for the room will guide you as you
make decisions about what to put in it.

Jakob and Collier (2014) produced guidance for people creating
sensory rooms for individuals with dementia. This is a great starting
point for some of the practical considerations of creating sensory

rooms, especially if you work in a care setting. This guidance is available to download for free online.

Converting a whole room or even a section of a room into a sensory room can be a big undertaking and will not be practical or possible for everyone. Here we consider some smaller improvised sensory environments which can have the same impact as the larger environments but do not place such a big demand on us as we create them.

Umbrellas

Sensory umbrellas are a mainstay of sensory engagement work, made popular by Flo Longhorn and Richard Hirstwood in the 1980s. Their popularity is buoyed along by their marvellous versatility and easiness to use. All you need is an umbrella. But first you need to get over any superstitions you may have about opening umbrellas inside. I have been doing it for years and I have survived so far without waves of bad luck coming my way!

Just popping up an umbrella and holding it above and slightly in front of you as you sit side by side in conversation with a person is enough to create a little private space. The canopy of the umbrella shields other faces and distractions from view and acts as a gentle deflector of sound.

There are a spectacular array of different styles and designs of umbrella available, from huge golfing umbrellas, to those that come down around the head and shoulders, you can even buy one with a clip on section that reaches to the floor – more of a portable tent than an umbrella. Patterns abound: I have a beautiful summer sky one printed with clouds and another with a galaxy set against the dark night sky. There are ones with animals, bright patterns, see through ones (draw on your own pattern with marker pens), beautifully ornate ones, ones with parts that light up, parasols – the list goes on and on. A good umbrella can be a sensory conversation in itself. However you may wish to do more...

An umbrella can be used as a stage for a rotating sensory conversation. Use the prongs that hold out the fabric of the umbrella as supports for a few small sensory resources. By clipping or tying things onto the umbrella you can add topics to your sensory conversation. You can even use a small set of battery-operated fairy lights to add twinkle to your umbrella. Ribbons dangling down can create a small world into which the two of you (yourself and your sensory conversation partner) can slip. If you are sharing sensory conversations with several people you can easily carry the umbrella from one to another, dipping it over them and giving them your full attention when it is their turn in the conversation. To see ideas for different umbrellas please visit The Sensory Projects website and follow the links to Facebook where my public photo albums are full of sensory wonders.

A hula hoop hidey hole

Having a little space to hide away in can be very soothing – the option to escape the world as you know it for a moment or two and enter a different space is very pleasurable. Hula hoop hidey holes are perfect for this. To make one you just need a large plastic hula hoop and a shower curtain. These can both be purchased inexpensively. If you want to get adventurous many companies now produce shower curtains printed with different scenes on them (e.g. a forest or an underwater scene). These are a little more expensive but work brilliantly for creating an environment.

Simply clip the shower curtain around the hula hoop as though it were the curtain rail in the bathroom and then tie cord across the hoop to allow it to be suspended. You can add further decoration by winding fairy lights around the hoop or draping lightweight fabric over it to create a roof. If you use a plain curtain you can project lights or pictures onto the outside so that the person inside can enjoy them. Adding gentle music to this set up provides another layer of sensory immersion. The first case study in Section 3 was inspired by hoop work. If you want to create a slightly larger space, hook the shower curtain to three or four coat hangers and hook these from different points to mark out a space.

Screens

In group environments it is often difficult to experience time alone. Time contentedly alone is as good for our mental wellbeing as well as time spent socially with others. Many people with dementia need constant supervision and to leave them truly on their own would not be wise. Nevertheless we can use screens, large boxes or curtains to give them a sense of privacy and to create a small sensory environment that allows them to rest from social interaction.

Padded display board screens are super for creating zones in a group setting as they not only screen off people visually from one another but their padding also absorbs sound, creating some auditory privacy as well. Namazi and Johnson (1992) found simply hanging cloth partitions reduced distractions among residents of a care home for people with dementia and contributed to their increased interest in an activity.

Someone who is seated can feel screened off if their line of sight is blocked; something really simple like a large cardboard box cut in half and weighted on a table top can do this, and the cardboard will also absorb some sound, creating a more secure-feeling auditory environment for the person within the space. You could decorate the inside of the box with photos from their life, or photos of beautiful scenery or images that might provoke their curiosity. For example, for someone with a background in engineering a picture of parts of a motor could be engaging.

Considering the pre existing sensory environments

When thinking about providing a sensory environment for a person with dementia it can be worth thinking through the different spaces currently on offer to them. Consider the different rooms available to them where they live and mentally do a sensory audit of them yourself. What can be heard in the rooms? What is the light like in the rooms? What smells are in the rooms?

When caring for an individual who, for example, is less mobile than they used to be we tend to seat them in the room we think of as being for sitting in (e.g. a living room or similar). These rooms are often spacious, bright and airy and have additional stimuli such as televisions or radios within them. For the person you care for this room could be the perfect place, but it could also not be. Televisions and radios may provide entertainment to those of us who enjoy good sensory functioning but for people experiencing a degree of sensory confusion they can actually be a drain on their ability to process information rather than a source of enjoyment. The presence of a television or radio that is always on can mean a person is less able to take in other environmental stimulation, and many care settings are already lacking in stimulation. Cohen and Weisman (1991) say that sensory deprivation has been identified as a potential problem in many dementia care environments.

The person you care for may prefer to sit in their shed, where the light is darker, the smell mustier, the sounds less synthetic and more natural. The person you care for may enjoy sitting in a bay window with the curtain drawn around them. I have even known people to hide under the stairs. Their relatives' interpretation was that they had got lost in the house, gone through the wrong door and got stuck, but when it happened repeatedly we reflected that it could be they were seeking out the smallest room in the house where they felt most secure. Of course I am not advising anyone to shut the person they care for up underneath the stairs and indeed when considering small spaces such as cupboards under stairs we need to be very careful to ensure there is sufficient air flow for someone who may want to stay in there for a few hours. But with simple preparations, perhaps a doorstop in the door to prevent it from closing fully, and with regular checks to make sure a person is okay, then it is perfectly possible to allow a person to spend their time where they feel safe rather than where convention dictates they should be.

One wonderful and much overlooked sensory space is the garden. Hussein (2010) looked at how a sensory garden could be just as effective a tool as a sensory room in the support of individuals with profound disabilities. If you are fortunate enough to have a garden or have access to a public garden it is likely that all the sensory stimuli you could want are already in place and the challenge will not be one of creating the environment but of enabling access. This could involve sorting out paving that is easy for the person you support to navigate, or making sure they have clothing that will allow them to sit out for as long as they like in the weather of the season. Do not automatically assume that rain means a person should be inside. Rain as a sensation is a delight – instead of bundling them inside stop for a moment yourself and feel how gentle it is on your skin; try not to worry about getting wet, so long as you have the capacity to dry off and you are not getting unpleasantly cold embrace the experience. Live the sensory moment; it is good for you!

Nina Ockenden-Powell blogs at Wild Happy Well about the mental health benefits of natural experiences, here she explains what natural environments have to offer individuals with dementia:

> The natural world is the environment within which we, as human beings, have evolved. Our senses are tuned into the colours, textures, sounds and other physical sensations nature provides. Our brains find the attributes of natural scenes inherently comforting (whereas urban scenes can cause discomfort). In other words, all of us humans, whatever our abilities or requirements, are hardwired to interact with nature through whichever of our senses work. There is a lot of scientific evidence that shows how interacting with nature and bringing it into our daily lives improves mental and physical health, irrespective of health condition or ability.
>
> For people with dementia nature can be used as a form of therapy to improve wellbeing in multiple ways. This can include spending time outside in nature, physically interacting with nature (e.g. gardening), or even viewing nature through a window. Nature reduces stress, improves mood, calms and relaxes people, and increases self-esteem and confidence. The effects can manifest immediately as well as longer term, meaning that if someone is experiencing a form of crisis, interacting with nature can provide immediate relief and calm from the situation/episode to help regain control of the emotions. Spending time in nature and interacting with it, even through simple tasks, can help create and bring back happy memories of time spent outside in the past. This may be particularly relevant for people with dementia

in bringing reassurance and a renewed sense of self as well as increased confidence. Nature can also act as a facilitator of social interaction which is important in dementia: chatting in a garden, helping with gardening tasks, or even looking out of the window together noticing the trees and birds can help people connect with each other via the calming medium of nature.

Nature is a truly multisensory experience which can be incredibly valuable for dementia patients. One of the best aspects of natural environments as sensory experiences is that the stimulation is typically very gentle, and overstimulation is avoided as excitation of one sense is often tempered by gentle stimulation of others. For example, when visiting a woodland, trees provide a strong visual stimulus, but this may be tempered by the rustling of the leaves, the delight and surprise of birdsong, sensations of bracken underfoot or hands touching bark. Taking the time to notice the changes in a garden, notice wildlife, or the changing of the seasons are excellent ways to connect with and bring nature into our daily lives and socialise with others. These simple approaches provide a multitude of ways to engage the senses in gentle, holistic ways that can stimulate the memory, calm the emotions, and enable social interactions. It is very easy to develop natural multisensory experiences on even the smallest scale: a herb garden is perfect! Simple planting can provide changing visual stimuli throughout the year from plants that are edible, smell wonderful and provide a variety of tactile sensations.

The wider world

As well as creating and becoming aware of sensory environments at home consider the sensory environments you ask a person with dementia to interact with. A trip, for example, to a shopping centre, a train station, or a hospital all require a person to cope with a very distinct sensory environment. Furthermore, these environments are liable to be different from their home environment where they feel safest.

Day *et al.* (2000) report that people with dementia often experience difficulties with sensory overstimulation, which may increase the agitation and confusion associated with dementia. If you feel a person you are supporting struggles with a particular sensory environment, but it is one where they must go (e.g. a hospital), consider taking some form of sensory support with you (e.g. ear muffs to block out noise, a fiddle mitt to provide a comforting distraction, something sweet to chew on – chewing and sweetness are both naturally soothing). Young *et al.* (2011) found that sensory stories can support people with profound intellectual disabilities to cope with sensitive issues (e.g. a trip to the dentist). They did this by incorporating the experiences of the event in a sensory story which could be shared multiple times together prior to the event, essentially practicing the experiences in a safe and reassuring environment.

Thinking about the sensory nature of the different environments a person with dementia is expected to interact with can give us an extra window through which to view their behaviour. Once you recognise something as a sensory problem you can look for sensory solutions to it where other solutions may not be working.

Summary: sensory environments

Creating small space sensory environments for an individual with dementia can help them to feel safe and encourage their engagement with activities. Considering larger environments such as gardens or shopping centres and the sensory properties they hold can help you provide therapeutic experiences to a person with dementia. This can also help you to understand why their behaviour may change in different situations whilst also giving you insight into how you can help them cope.

Section 8

Sensory support for mental wellbeing

Orientation

Simple considerations of how we select stimuli and facilitate sensory experiences can have a profound effect on the mental wellbeing of the person we are supporting. A person experiencing mental ill health will often become disengaged so the very act of sensory engagement itself can be beneficial. Well-chosen sensory activities can provide stimulation which increases awareness and attention in people with dementia (Jakob and Collier 2014). The use of multisensory environments could support people with dementia who are also suffering from anxiety or low mood (Hope 1998). Sensory activities can reduce agitation in people with dementia in care environments (Livingston *et al.* 2014). In addition to the above considering how the facilitation of sensory experiences can contribute to a person's understanding of fundamental concepts that underpin mental wellbeing (e.g. Time, Change, Agency and Self), also enables us to promote their mental wellbeing through the use of simple sensory strategies.

In all situations, whether you are telling someone an elaborate sensory story, taking them into an immersive multisensory environment or simply handing over a sensory item, facilitation is key. How we facilitate a sensory experience is what makes the difference between that experience having a positive or negative effect. In this chapter we are going to look at the very simplest of experiences and how our facilitation of these effects the mental wellbeing of those we support. I have used simple experiences as the example in order that we might focus solely on the facilitation and not get distracted by a new weird and wonderful sensory idea, but of course how we facilitate those more complex sensory experiences also has an impact on mental wellbeing.

Physical ill health comes in many forms, there are a plethora of diseases and infections we can catch, of injuries we can do ourselves and conditions we acquire. However, despite the great diversity of illnesses available to us there is a lot of common ground between the lived experience of these illnesses. Were we to ask sufferers of different conditions how they feel they would likely report similar things: feelings of pain, of aching, tiredness, a lack of appetite, and so on.

Mental ill health is the same as physical ill health in that it comes in many forms but that those different forms share common ground when it comes to the lived experience of having them. People suffering from mental ill health are likely to feel anxious and insecure; they turn inward and close themselves off from the world, or defend themselves violently from it and so on. When we delve further into the similarities in experience we find that many forms of mental ill health are underpinned by the same fundamental beliefs.

In this section I am going to take five factors that I believe underpin a wide range of conditions of mental ill health and look at how our facilitation of sensory experience can address each one.

Engagement

Engagement comes top of the list when we look at links between sensory experience and mental health. Someone who is experiencing mental ill health is likely to become disengaged from their sensory experience. There is a tendency to turn inwards, to self reflection, to worries circling in the mind, and close off those avenues we have to outer experience: our senses.

People experiencing mental ill health may lose their appetite, and they may withdraw from activities they used to enjoy; people with chronic depression often stay in bed, or in a single chair, limiting their sensory experience of the world still further.

Sadly, but unsurprisingly, this is a two-way street and mental ill health can actually effect our physical capacity to engage with the world. For example, people suffering from depression lose some of their ability to smell and so are less able to access the olfactory world.

If we can engage people with sensory experience then we are a part of turning that inward looking mind outward again. Engagement with the world around you (e.g. noticing the bird-song, smelling the roses, wanting tactile experience, pleasure in food, delight in music) is a sign of good mental health and works to promote mental health.

A lack of engagement with sensory experience can be a warning sign of mental ill health. A disengaged person may appear passive and unresponsive, they may talk less than they once did, seem less animated. If you are someone who knows them well then you will know what they are typically like and be able to spot the signs of decreasing engagement. Sadly a decrease in interest in the world is often assumed to be a natural part of dementia, and other conditions, and so is viewed as 'normal under the circumstances'. To hold the idea that mental ill health is normal and to be expected is very dangerous to the wellbeing of those being supported.

A lack of engagement with the sensory world caused by a mental health condition can also manifest itself in violence. A person who is feeling insecure, down, frightened, anxious, may try to retire to a place of low stimulation. Imagine a frightened animal taking themselves into a small, dark hole to hide from the monsters they imagine are coming. If we reach into that hole to encourage that scared little animal they are likely to bite our hand or scratch us because they are so very frightened. The person you support does not look like a cute cowering mouse, they look like the person you used to know, and when they lash out it is not the mouse scratch or nip of my metaphor; it is a smack or a punch and it looks like what they would have looked like if they were angry; if they were unpleasant, or unkind. It can be hard for us to see these actions and understand them through the lens of the condition and the co-occurring mental health problems. These actions look so very similar to something we would have once despised that it's hard to see them as the actions of fear, but this is what we must do.

Dementia very often co-occurs with mental health conditions, particularly depression, but it does not *necessarily* cause these. It is possible to have dementia without depression and this is what sensory engagement work aims for. Spaull *et al.* (1998) found observable changes in levels of interaction, active looking and interest in patients with dementia sharing sensory exchanges with a facilitator.

A good facilitator can support someone experiencing mental ill health to become engaged in their sensory world. That engagement in the sensory world invites their attention outwards and counters the mental ill health they are experiencing.

How do you do this? How do you engage someone whose mental health is causing them to turn their attention inwards?

First, you need to choose a wonderful experience, one that is likely to interest them. Remember a time when you were ill and off your food, when you started to feel better what was the food that you were willing to eat – was it something very bland and gentle, or was it a treat food? Depending on the circumstances, it might have been either of these. It is these sorts of experiences that you are looking for.

A sensory experience that is an utter delight, such a treat that you would not want to turn away from it, might tempt you out of your confinement. (Think of the little animal cowering in the hole, it is the tasty piece of cheese that lures them back out).

Alternatively a sensory experience so gentle that it is a stepping stone out of confinement might be what's needed. Something that feels very nearly like the hiding place where the person felt safe but is just a fraction more outward. Maybe you had a migrane and shut the curtains to block out the light, then when you began to feel better you cracked them open just a little. This is what we are looking for.

The information in Section 4 will help you as you think about what sorts of experiences to choose. If you want further information on what sorts of experiences would be likely to work my book *Sensory-being for Sensory Beings* provides more extensive explanations.

Once you have chosen your stimulus then you need to facilitate it sensitively. This will be offering it slowly, not forcing it upon someone. It may just mean leaving it near them for them to encounter and explore as they wish. It might mean leaving it around for days, even weeks, before they show an interest. Their frightened cowering spirit will only hunker down more if you approach in boisterous ways and expect quick responses. Tread softly, be near, touch compassionately, understand their resistance, even their violence as fear, show them the beauty of the sensory world again.

Time

An understanding of time and its progression is a vital part of mental health. When we have a sense of time moving on, we have a sense of progress. When we know that time moves, that there is now and that there is something after now, there is next, then we can anticipate a time when things are different. Time is one of the fundamental components of hope, and hopeful is how mentally healthy people feel.

Time is also a very tricky abstract concept. Time is not something we can see or lay our hands upon. It is hard to explain and it is easy to get muddled about it, especially if you have a condition like dementia that is affecting your mental capacity.

Offering the person you are supporting sensory experiences that reinforce notions of time is a way of supporting them at a fundamental level to retain their ability to hope.

A very simple way to offer sensory experiences that reinforce notions of time is to use sensory strings – described in Section 4 – consistently. If the person you are supporting regularly encounters a sensory string they will be supported in retaining an understanding of how that string works; that when they encounter one item on the string they know there is another one after that, and another after that. The string becomes a representation of the sequence of time. And for as long as they are able to reach for the next item they hold onto their awareness that there is a next. Knowing that there is a next is key to understanding that things can be different, key to feeling hope, key to optimism.

Your facilitation of the string is important as you seek to support all those wonderful things mentioned above. As you share a sensory string with someone you are not going to unclip and bring things forwards to show them – doing this is like shuffling time; it makes things more confused. You are going to display the string in the same way every time, possibly using the same string to show different resources. By keeping the experience of the string itself consistent you help the person you are supporting to maintain their understanding of it. You will help them to move from one item on the string to the next, at a pace that suits them. You will be alert to the possibility that one day they will become stuck on the experience they are on and may need help to move to the next one. When they are no longer able to move along the string themselves you will move it slowly for them so that their senses are still told about the progression of time.

I have used the example of a sensory string as it was one of the resources we have looked at in this book, but strings are not the only way of reinforcing notions of time. Time at its essence is sequence so any activities that hold a sequence within them will be supportive of notions of time. For example, books with their beginnings, middles and ends, sensory stories, boxes that open, reveal something and then close, and meditation beads, prayer beads or rosaries that people are used to moving through their fingers, bead by bead. As you assess the sensory experiences you might offer to someone ask yourself whether they have an opportunity to experience sequence within them, and if they do then you know you have found something that will be good for supporting someone to feel hope.

Change

Underpinning many feelings of mental ill health is the idea that things will not change and cannot be changed by the individual. Depression, for example, is underpinned by a combination of time and change. The depressed person feels that they will feel this way forever; that their depressed state will never change.

The possibility for change and the ability to instigate change are preventative of feelings concerning the impossibility of change and the inevitability of one's current predicament. In many very simple ways we can give people the opportunity to experience and cause change in a sensory way.

As you select sensory resources to support awareness of change think about experiences that demonstrate change (e.g. lights that change colour) but also, and in many ways better, experiences in which the experiencer can cause change. A very simple example of this is the metallic space blankets often used to wrap marathon runners up in once they have finished their marathon. These foil blankets are a very inexpensive resource but the capacity for change in the experience is huge. By touching them and moving just a little an experiencer causes a change in their sound environment as well as a change in their visual environment. They are wonderfully responsive.

Another great example of the opportunity to experience change is the knocking down of a tower of bricks or plastic cups. Young children enjoy this precisely because the impact their small gesture has is so huge. At first the bricks are neatly stacked and ordered and stationary – they push one and suddenly there is noise, there is movement and there is a visual jumble. How wonderful! If the person you are supporting enjoys this too then you are onto a winner. However it is worth being cautious: some people with dementia who are experiencing the world in a sensory way may retain notions of it being wrong to knock things over; they may feel panic at the thought of something falling, fear getting in trouble for making a mess. It maybe that with your attentive and joyful facilitation they are soon engaged in the game of knocking things over. But it maybe that you are looking for alternatives, games like Jenga where knocking things down is a part of the game may be more accessible, or, for a really satisfying activity that you can share together, invest in some coloured dominos and set up domino rallies for them to knock down. To make this activity even more beautiful and visually inviting buy transparent coloured dominos and set up the rallies somewhere where sunlight can fall on them. Engaging in activities like this together is a chance for you both to feel focused and engaged and calm, which is good for your mental wellbeing as well as the mental wellbeing of the person you are supporting. If you are interested in finding out more about shared sensory experiences to support mental wellbeing my book *Sensory-being for Sensory Beings* has further examples.

Agency

When we are feeling mentally healthy we feel we have control over our lives and can change things that trouble us. To have this control taken away from us is very distressing: we use the removal of control over one's life as a form of punishment for criminals. You have probably experienced situations of illness where you had to relinquish control of your life for a while, perhaps letting someone help you or handing over responsibilities that were yours to someone else. We are grateful towards those who help when we need it but we do not like giving up control. Giving up control often leaves us feeling powerless, helpless and insecure.

The person you are supporting has probably had to give up a lot of control over their life, and has had control taken from them when they were no longer able to exert it effectively. They may not be able to identify what it was that they once did but can no longer do, but even without the knowledge as to what the control was they will have that sense of control not being theirs, of things being out of their hands.

There are two key sensory things we can do when it comes to supporting someone who is feeling a lack of control. One is to make them feel safe and the other is to offer them experiences that have agency within them.

To support someone in feeling safe in a sensory way we need to enable them to process and understand the information they are getting from their senses. This may mean that we need to restrict information so that there is not too much for them to process. Loud, busy environments can be very difficult and can heighten that sense of a loss of control. In contract a smaller, calmer, quieter environment can be more comforting. Often times we support people by doing what we would want were we in their situation; that is a lovely start point to begin from, but it is important that we recognise our differences as we do this. For example, I myself, if I were ill, would want to be curled up on the sofa watching television with the curtains drawn. In the main this is also an experience that would support someone accessing the world in a sensory way. Drawing the curtains reduces the pressure of sight in the room; hiding on the sofa creates a small enclosed environment that is naturally soothing. However the television is only comforting to me because I can process what is going on. If you look at the world presented by the television it is loud and vibrant and busy and full of different things, exactly the sort of environment you are looking to avoid. If the person you are supporting cannot access television in a meaningful way, if their eyes do not pick out the characters, their ears do not follow the speech, their mind does not keep up with the ever changing narratives, then a television is just a drain on sensory abilities. Television is just one example, others could include having the radio on, or being in a room with lots of pattern or having different plug-in scent diffusers around the house. Think about things in a purely sensory way; put yourself in their situation and think through each of your senses in turn: what am I hearing here, what can I smell here, and so on. Identify places of low and high stimulation and to comfort someone take them to somewhere offering low levels of stimulation.

Offering sensory support to feeling safe is step one when using sensory engagement strategies to support someone who is feeling out of control. Someone who does not feel safe will not engage, so you will always look to make sure the person you are supporting feels secure in their environment before you offer them any form of sensory stimuli to engage with. Once you are confident you have enabled them to feel as safe as they can you can then begin to offer them sensory experiences that support their agency to counter their feelings of lack of control.

Sensory experiences containing the opportunity for agency within them give people the chance to feel their own power again and to exert control over their surroundings. Accessing experiences which offer you control is a way of getting rid of those out of control feelings.

A sensory experience has agency within it if it happens in some way because of you. So, for example, the foil blanket described above would be perfect because the sound and the shifting visuals happen because the person exploring it moves. Although the sensory stimulation gained is the same if the facilitator moves the blanket (e.g. the same sounds are produced, the same change in visual experience happens) the mental wellbeing of the experiencer is only reinforced if they are the active agent within the experience, i.e. if they move the blanket. Sometimes it can be very tempting to do things for a person, to show them the outcome that will happen if bells are rung, or foil blankets scrunched, etc., but hold back. Show interest in the experience, demonstrate that you expect it to happen, wait with baited breath, focus your eyes, lean in and so on, but resist the temptation to *do*. Allow the person you are supporting to be the one who does the doing; allow them to be the active agent in the activity. In this way you give them power; you give them control. You may only be able to give them tiny bits of control throughout the day, for their own safety you need to be in control of certain things, but where it is safe to do so give them control and do so at every possible opportunity. Think of it as being like feeding their body to keep them physically healthy – you are feeding their mind to keep them mentally healthy. Where once their mind would have accessed large meals of control when they took big decisions about their own life and the lives of others, now all it can manage is control the size of a grain of rice, but the hunger is the same so they will need a great many grains of rice in order to feel sated. Look for experiences you can offer them that in some way happen because of them and in these you gift them agency.

Self

The final concept that I want to look at with regard to ideas that underpin our mental wellbeing is our sense of self. Caught up in this is an idea of who we are and what we are worth; it is the thought of our very 'I-ness'. Consider a time when you have felt great about life and your prospects within it, your idea of who you are, your sense of self: your 'I-ness' is large, it expands with your joy and hope. It is as if your 'I' gets bigger. Contrastingly think of a time when you felt low, frightened, weak, pessimistic – correspondingly your sense of self shrinks: the power you think of yourself as having lessens, your grasp on control weakens and your 'I-ness' whimpers in the corner. We speak of feeling 'very small', and this is what happens to your sense of self when you are experiencing mental ill health.

Any sensory resource that enables a person to know their own presence in the world and to declare it reinforces that sense of 'I-ness' of self. You are looking for experiences that let them know they are here and enable them to let everyone else know they are here. Examples of such experiences would be: mirrors, bracelets with bells on, microphones or small recording devices, paint and the opportunity to make marks with it, and the space to dance with music to dance to.

You may have noticed that there is a lot of overlap with what we are looking for when we look for sensory experiences to address mental wellbeing – how wonderful that this is the case! With a simple resource like a foil blanket we can allow someone to know they are there: the blanket makes a noise and tells them they moved, it is saying 'You are there, you did something' and that reinforces their sense of self, allows them agency, teaches them about change, and if they repeat the movement they declare themselves and their capabilities to the world. All of that from foil blanket! It is not the case that every sensory resource does all of these things; for example, a sequence string does not necessarily hold opportunity for change within it (but it could). The value in considering things according to these different criteria does not come from making sets of resources to address each one. These different criteria are merely different windows we can look through when selecting sensory resources and each window has the potential to show us slightly different resources and lead us in different ways to look for those resources. The most important thing these windows do is remind us just how important these simple resources are to the person we support.

The wonderful thing about sensory engagement work is that with a resource you might previously have overlooked you can engage someone's senses, support their wellbeing and your own, exercise their cognitive faculties, share a connection, tell a story, offer safety and from time to time you may even prompt a memory or two. I hope you are able to take the arising of the person you support's need for sensory stimulation as an invitation to explore together, and I hope you discover many wonderful things as you share the sensory stories and conversations together. My very best wishes for your continuing sensory adventures.

Summary: sensory support for mental wellbeing

Sensory engagement itself is good for mental wellbeing, for individuals with dementia and for the rest of the population. As you engage in sensory exchanges with the person you support, you benefit the mental health of all involved. Concepts of time, change, agency and self fundamentally underpin our mental wellbeing, without these being reinforced we can quickly become lost. Simple sensory strategies can be employed to support the mental wellbeing of individuals with dementia.

Section 9

Conclusion

Dementia is a cruel disease, taking what we have known of our loved ones from us whilst they are still with us. The confusion, distress, violence and disability that come with it are hard enough for loved ones to witness, let alone to cope with and manage. But even within such a devastating disease people find moments of light.

Caring for a person with dementia, whether personally or professionally, is hard. People often feel guilty for struggling with what can be a difficult task. Finding a difficult task difficult is not an indication of failing, merely a reflection of life as it is. The guilt is not your own failing but a desire to be able to do more, which is an admirable thing to have. Trust your instincts, they will often be right. But do not be misled by the temptation to interpret words and behaviour to mean what they would have meant before dementia came into play. A person may shout 'go away' at you, meaning to communicate to you, the person nearest them, the person most trusted, that they want the confusion they are experiencing to go away. A person may lash out and hit you, not through a desire to harm you but because they are afraid and need to defend themselves.

By considering behaviour, communication and responses through a sensory lens we give ourselves an extra layer of understanding that we can use to sensitively support those in our care. Through this book we have explored various ways to use sensory experiences to build connections, facilitate independence, support someone in feeling safe, and enrich and add enjoyment to life. Because dementia has such a profound effect on a person's memory the tendency with support strategies is to focus on preserving and recovering memories. As much as we may long to do this, ultimately we will ultimately be unable to hold back the tide that takes those things from us. By shifting the focus from connection with memories to connection with the person as they are now we can take some of the pressure off both the individual experiencing the condition and ourselves and find ways to stay with our loved ones as they progress through their experience of dementia.

We may long to be able to connect and communicate with them in the ways that we did before, or in the ways that are normal to us, and not being able to so is disheartening. When we seek instead to have sensory conversations we open up the possibility of connecting with them as they are now. People can at first find it strange to be having sensory conversations with a loved one they once had verbal conversations with. Playing with toys and sensory resources can feel remote to them, the loved one who used to be so sharp in their conversations fading even in their memories as they interact together. This is where we need to be conscious of the meaningfulness of sensory exchanges. No, you will not be having a conversation about politics, or philosophy; it will not be a conversation that maps neatly onto words. But as you reach for it to do this, as you look for the yes's and the no's and the verbalised memories you are trying to enforce a linguistic view of the world. Meaning is not word based. Look again.

When we manage to create a space of safety and trust in which a sensory conversation can flourish we see in a person's responses and interactions their heart, we see them bare of any facades they may have chosen to wear in the past, and we see their pure self. What a conversation to be having! How intimate, how personal, how precious. As with any conversation, word based or sensory based, it is the meaning behind what we say that matters. In words we may choose the wrong ones but a loved one will understand us anyway because they know our meaning. With sensory conversations we may be sharing a child's toy or a scrap of chain from a DIY store; it does not matter, what matters is the meaning within the exchange. It is the closeness, the shared experience, the connection – and those things can be accessed with childish items or adult items, with wildly expensive items or with fantastically cheap items. Once you feel the meaning in a sensory conversation you will feel deeply privileged when someone chooses to share one with you. You may even find it relaxing to be let off the hook of having to find the right words all the time. Let words and time drift away; be there in the moment with that person and that experience, and treasure the *now*.

Dementia may take many things from you and your loved one, but in sensory experiences you can share a connection together until the end. My very best wishes for your journey together.

Appendix

Do I actually need to physically intervene? Is it absolutely necessary?

Are there alternatives available such as speaking to de-escalate? Containing rather than restraining or even just waiting until a more opportune moment where all parties have clearer thoughts and are perhaps calmer? If objects are being thrown or if items in a classroom are in the way are we able to risk assess the environment to make it a safer place?

When it is deemed as necessary to support, hold, guide or assist someone to release, perhaps it will usually come about where there are one of three reasons:

1. to prevent harm to oneself

2. to prevent harm to others and

3. to prevent damage to property (which often falls in line with preventing harm to ones, self or others, I find).

If it is necessary to intervene then the second test is about how much force is used and the term used is proportionate.

The force used must be equal or less to the harm (or perceived harm) to be avoided

Meaning: If we cause discomfort or harm that is greater than which we were avoiding in the first place then the use of force would be disproportionate and therefore deemed unreasonable.

In many cases holding a limb, guiding a person's arms away or supporting someone who is frustrated through a period of turbulence or distress can be vital skills that staff and carers often learn as they go along – if there is a need it is often a good idea for training to be sourced that fits the bill for their individual requirements.

References

Baker, R. *et al.* (2001) 'A randomized controlled trial of the effects of multi-sensory stimulation (MSS) for people with dementia.' *British Journal of Clinical Psychology 40*, 81–96.

Behrman, S. *et al.* (2014) 'Considering the senses in the diagnosis and management of dementia.' *Sophie Maturitas 77*, 305–310.

Bower, H.M. (1967). 'Sensory stimulation and the treatment of senile dementia.' *Medical Journal of Australia 1*, 1113–1119.

Canevelli, M. *et al.* (2017) 'Inappropriate sexual behaviors among community-dwelling patients with dementia.' *Am J Geriatr Psychiatry 25*, 4, 365–371.

Cohen, U. and Weisman, G.D. (1991) *Holding On To Home: Designing Environments For People With Dementia.* Baltimore: Johns Hopkins University Press.

Day, K *et al.* (2000) 'The therapeutic design of environments for people with dementia: a review of the empirical research.' *The Gerontologist 40*, 4, 397–416.

Epel, E. *et al.* (2009) 'Can meditation slow the rate of cellular aging? Cognitive stress, mindfulness and telomeres.' *Annals of the New York Academy of Sciences 1172*, 34–53: www.ncbi.nlm.nih.gov/pmc/articles/PMC3057175

Gerlach, L. and Kales, H. (2017) 'Learning their language: the importance of detecting and managing pain in dementia.' *Am J Geriatr Psychiatry 25*, 2, 155–157.

Grace, J. (2014) *Sensory Stories for Children and Teens with Special Educational Needs.* London: Jessica Kingsley Publishers.

Grace and Silva (2017) 'Refining the guidance for sensory story telling with individuals with PMLD: a move towards improved research and practice.' PMLD Link 29, 88, 11–14: www.thesensoryprojects.co.uk/sensory-stories

Grace, J. (2017) *Sensory-Being for Sensory Beings.* London: Routledge.

Hope, K.W. (1998) 'The effects of multisensory environments on older people with dementia.' *Journal of Psychiatric and Mental Health Nursing 5*, 377–385.

Hussein, H. (2010) 'Using the sensory garden as a tool to enhance the educational development and social interaction of children with special needs.' *Support for Learning 25*, 1, 24–31.

Jakob, A. and Collier, L. (2014) *How To Make a Sensory Room for People Living With Dementia: A Guide Book.* London: Kingston University.

Kindell, J. *et al.* (2014) 'Life story resources in dementia care: a review.' *Quality in Ageing and Older Adults 15*, 3, 151–161.

Kulkarni, A. *et al.* (2010) 'Massage and touch therapy in neonates: the current evidence.' *Indian Paediatrics 47*, 771–776. Accessed 21 December 2017 at http://medind.nic.in/ibv/t10/i9/ibvt10i9p771.pdf

Lacey, P. (2006) 'Inclusive Literacy.' *PMLD Link 18*, 3, 55, 11–13.

Lambe, L. and Hogg, J. (2013) 'Sensitive Stories: Tackling Challenges for People with Profound Intellectual Disabilities through Multisensory Storytelling.' In N. Grove (2013) *Using Storytelling to Support Children and Adults with Special Needs*. Abingdon: Routledge.

Leighton, R. Oddy, C. and Grace, J. (2016) 'Using sensory stories with individuals with dementia.' *The Journal of Dementia Care 24*, 4, 28–31.

Livingston, G. *et al.* (2014) 'A systematic review of the clinical effectiveness and cost-effectiveness of sensory, psychological and behavioural interventions for managing agitation in older adults with dementia.' *Health Technol Assess 18*, 39.

Longhorn, F. (2008) *The Sensology Workout*. Flo Longhorn Publications.

McKeown, J. *et al.* (2015) 'You have to be mindful of whose story it is: The challenges of undertaking life story work with people with dementia and their family carers.' *Dementia 14*, 2, 238–256.

Maslow, A. (1943) 'A theory of human motivation.' *Psychological Review* 50, 4, 370–396.

Namazi, K.H. and Johnson, B. D. (1992). 'The effects of environmental barriers on the attention span of Alzheimer's disease patients.' *American Journal of Alzheimer's Care and Related Disorders and Research 7*, 9–15.

NICE (2006) 'Dementia: supporting people with dementia and their carers in health and social care.' *Clinical guidelines CG42*, Sections: 1.7.1.2. and 1.8.1.3.

Onishi, J. *et al.* (2006) 'Behavioral, psychological and physical symptoms in group homes for older adults with dementia. *Int Psychogeriatr 18*, 75–86.

PAMIS (2002) Real Lives: Real Stories, summary of results leaflet. University of Dundee.

Penne, A. *et al.* (2012) 'Staff interactive style during multisensory storytelling with persons with profound intellectual and multiple disabilities.' *Journal of Intellectual Disability Research 56*, 167–178.

Preece, D. and Zhao, Y. (2014) *An evaluation of Bag Books multi-sensory stories*. Northampton: The University of Northampton.

Provine, R. (2000) *Laughter: A Scientific Investigation*. London: Penguin Books.

Sheil, K. (2016) 'Sensory stories: what does the literature tell us?' *SLD Experience 74*, 1, 6–9.

Spaull, D., Leach, C. and Frampton, I. (1998) 'An evaluation of the effects of sensory stimulation with people who have dementia.' *Behavioural and Cognitive Psychotherapy*, Cambridge University Press, 26, 77–86

Taylor, J. (2006) 'Using multi sensory stories to develop literacy skills and to teach sensitive topics.' *PMLD Link 18*, 3, 55, 14–16.

Ten Brug *et al.* (2012) 'Multi-sensory storytelling for persons with profound intellectual and multiple disabilities: an analysis of the development, content and application.' *Practice Journal of Applied Research in Intellectual Disabilities 25*, 350–359.

Vlaskamp, C., Hiemstra, S.J. and Wiersma, L.A. (2007) 'Becoming aware of what you know or need to know: gathering client and context characteristics in day services for persons with profound intellectual and multiple disabilities.' *Journal of Policy and Practice in Intellectual Disabilities 4*, 2, 97–103.

Watson, M. (2002) *Developing Literacy Skills through Multi-sensory Story-telling in Children and Young Adults with Profound and Multiple Learning Disabilities*. Dundee: University of Dundee.

Young, H., Fenwick, M., Lambe, L. and Hogg, J. (2011) 'Multisensory storytelling as an aid to assisting people with profound intellectual disabilities to cope with sensitive issues: a multiple research methods analysis of engagement and outcomes.' *European Journal of Special Needs Education 26*, 2, 127–142.

Young, H. and Lambe, L. (2011) 'Multi sensory story telling for people with profound and multiple learning disabilities.' *PMLD Link 23*, 1, 68, 29–31.

Subject Index

Author Index